Been There...

Whatever eating problems you've had, we've had them too: sneak eating, binging, purging, compulsive exercise, or just forever fighting with the same ten or twenty pounds. Like you, over the years we have tried every diet and weight-loss program in search of the perfect formula to drop those extra pounds that were making our lives miserable.

Who Has Succeeded Using 7 Secrets of Slim People

- Anyone who regularly struggles with losing the last ten or so pounds.

- People who repeatedly cycle between overeating and restricting food.

- People who eat to alleviate emotions such as stress, sadness, anger, and anxiety.

- Compulsive overeaters.

- People who exercise obsessively.

- Health-conscious people who are exasperated by ever-contradictory nutritional and medical information about how to eat best.

- Mothers who want their children to be their natural weight and to be normal, healthy eaters.

- Adolescents, twelve to twenty years old, who are seeking peer approval and are compelled to match social standards of beauty and fitness.

- Mates, parents, or intimates of any of the above.

the Seven SECRETS of SLIM People

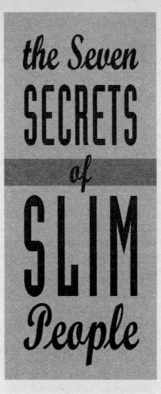

the Seven SECRETS of SLIM People

Vikki Hansen, MSW

Shawn Goodman

HarperPaperbacks
A Division of HarperCollinsPublishers

HarperPaperbacks
A Division of HarperCollins*Publishers*
10 East 53rd Street, New York, NY 10022-5299

HarperCollins®, ♣®, HarperPaperbacks™, are trademarks of
HarperCollins Publishers, Inc.

A hardcover edition of this book was published in 1997
by Hay House Inc.

First HarperPaperbacks printing: January 1998

Printed in the United States of America

Visit HarperPaperbacks on the World Wide Web at
http://www.harpercollins.com

❖ 10 9 8 7 6

To Dennis—the love of my life, without whom, love, a great life, and this book would not exist! And to Shawn, for your daily love and support which has smoothed out many of life's bumps and blows.

—VIKKI

To my family, who have been a constant source of love, support and hilarity. And to Vikki, for your lifelong devotion as my friend. (You didn't know it was for life, did you?)

—SHAWN

Vikki and Shawn wish to thank Marjorie Braman, Publishing Director, for her great vision and belief in this book; Carolyn Marino, Editorial Director, for her generous guidance and unerring eye; Jessica Lichtenstein, Senior Editor, for her perfect blend of creativity and pragmatism; Joe Wojak, for giving this book its auspicious beginning; and Leonida Karpik, Director of Publicity, for a fabulous job with the media.

Contents

- "I'm Afraid I'll Be Judged if I Eat Something Fattening, Since I'm Not Slim!"
- "Where does Exercise Fit In?"
- "I Feel Fat"
- "I'm Eating Just Like You've Said, and I'm Not Losing Weight"
- If You Have More Questions

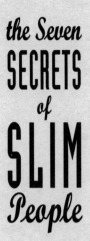

the Seven
SECRETS
of
SLIM
People

Preface

Shawn's Story

I never knew I had an eating problem. I just assumed everyone ate more or less the way I ate. I would polish off a box of Entenmann's cookies while I did my grocery shopping, before I even walked out of the market, and then fast the next day, followed by another day of Entenmann's. Another day, I would eat two heads of broccoli with lemon juice and half a chocolate cake. Meanwhile, I did aerobics and dance classes two hours a day, followed by Lifecycling or weight lifting. I never knew whether I was hungry or full. Instead, I blindly devoured everything fattening that I knew I wasn't supposed to eat and then punished myself with Draconian deprivation.

To this day, I can't believe I lived my life that way, in one form or another, since I was 13 and for the next 15 years. That's not a life. Yet, my eating habits weren't so different from any other female I knew from junior high school, through high school, college, and then into real life.

I became Vikki's first guinea pig as she developed an eating approach 18 years ago that completely and permanently changed my life. The Seven Secrets made me a normal eater. I get to eat anything I want, enjoy it, and be my perfect body size. And this is going on my 14th year! I have not dieted or deprived myself of one french fry or one banana split since then.

The deepest reward of this method cannot be measured simply in lost pounds or inches. The total freedom I discovered with food has created immeasurable freedom in every part of my life.

Vikki's Story

I struggled with food, weight, and body issues for 23 years. I was anorexic in high school, bulimic in college, and a compulsive eater, a yo-yo dieter, for the next 15 years. Although I lost and gained hundreds of pounds over those 23 years, mostly, I struggled with those "last 10 pounds" that I could never lose and KEEP OFF. I totally despaired of ever getting my eating permanently under control. I either felt temporary control while I was dieting or exercising like mad, or I was losing control and regaining the weight. Sound familiar? I was on every diet imaginable during that time, studied nutrition, and even became a therapist to try to solve my own weight problem. Nothing worked. Then, 13 years ago, I discovered how to be completely free from any struggle with food or weight. For the last 12 years, I have helped thousands of other people find freedom. I have lectured and conducted workshops all over the world.

This book is a compilation of all we have learned and taught with respect to food and eating. We've been fortunate enough to see many people discover an entirely new relationship with food and their bodies.

The Seven Secrets of Slim People is an important book in **The Joy of Living Series** of self-improvement books and materials. It has been inspired by the more than 80 percent of American women who have dieted in their lives and never found peace with eating and their bodies. This material has given both them and us final peace and liberation.

PROFESSIONAL PROFILES

Vikki Hansen, MSW, has founded and directed three eating disorder clinics. She is also a director of M.E.D.I.C.A. (Mood and Eating Disorder Institute of California), a nonprofit corporation formed for public education. Vikki is a widely acknowledged and respected expert in the field. She has lectured worldwide and given many presentations to professional organizations, including the prestigious American Psychological Association National Convention, and the American Association of Partial Hospitalization National Convention. She lives in Central California.

Shawn Goodman founded and directed a corporate marketing business in San Francisco and has been a print and television journalist. Shawn graduated magna cum laude with a B.A. in writing and literature from the University of Michigan, and has been a student of religious philosophy for ten years. She has also recovered from being a compulsive eater and exerciser.

Introduction

We've Been There

Whatever eating problem you've had, we've had them, too: sneak eating, binging, purging, compulsive dieting, compulsive exercise, or just forever fighting with the same ten or twenty pounds. Like you, over the years we have tried every diet and weight-loss program in search of the perfect formula to drop those extra pounds that were making our lives miserable.

This book is not only the product of clinical research and scientific theory. Every strategy in this book is born from our personal eating struggles over many years and from the struggles of thousands of people like yourself, with whom we have worked. Their needs have ranged from repeatedly trying to shed "those last few pounds," to those who have wanted to overcome severe, lifelong eating disorders. Most of their lives have been irreversibly changed. They are eating whatever they want in their ideal bodies and never feel out of control of their eating. They are our inspiration and our motivation, so we want to share this knowledge and wisdom with you in a simple, enjoyable way.

Most Diets and Diet Books Have Got It Wrong

Diets and diet books say that *weight* is the *problem* that needs to be solved. Weight is the *symptom*, not the problem. These books give you their newest hottest, "diet-of-the-minute" that often contradicts the last newest, hottest, "diet-of-the-minute." Follow their regime (i.e., eat *only* protein *or* carbohydrates *or* fruit and vegetables), they say, and you will lose weight. You may lose weight and you probably have lost weight on more than one diet. But, guess what? If weight alone were the *problem*, you would have to lose it only one time, and your problem would be solved forever.

Why This Book Is Different

Why is this book different from all of the other thousands of diet books that have been published? This book is radically different in three ways.

First, this book treats the CAUSES of overeating. Most other diets treat only the superficial *symptom* of excess weight. You do not want to lose weight *again*. You want to lose weight permanently. By simply and gently attacking the cause of overeating, you *permanently* solve the problem of excess weight. Our strategy is time-tested and proven. You will lose weight permanently—simply and gently.

Second, this way is so simple! We take all of the mystery out of eating normally, like slim people. You will truly be enjoying eating, and at the same time achieve your optimum health and most beautiful body. And you will do this without scales, calorie- or fat-gram counting, complicated food combining, or fanatical exercise regimens. The best part is that you already know how to eat, according to *The Seven Secrets*, without realizing it. This method is natural and automatic—you just need a refresher course.

Third, this approach gives you total freedom. Diets give you restrictive eating rules that may help you temporarily lose weight, so long as you continue to restrict your eating according to the diet. At some point, though (when you lose the weight or when the diet fails), you always go off the diet. However, this approach gives you permanent weight loss without any restrictive eating. There's no diet to "go off of." This method not only permanently frees you from your excess weight, but also frees you to completely enjoy eating whatever you want.

This approach leads you, one day at a time, through easily achievable, proven steps, toward the goal of your perfect body, and lifelong freedom from overeating and dieting.

The Written Exercises Are the Key to Success

We cannot urge you strongly enough to do the simple exercises in this book. They are absolutely the key to your success in permanently achieving your ideal body and for eliminating diets forever. They are exciting and will reveal surprising and comforting information about yourself. Above all, you already know from your own experience that the best way to learn something is to *DO IT*. The exercises are the fastest, surest, and easiest way to become a slim person.

You Can't Read This Book Too Many Times

We also recommend that you read the book twice or more. The information here, although simple, is very concentrated. Others who have succeeded using these secrets have read the material many times, and have enjoyed doing so. The better they know the material, the more familiar and confident they become about the life improvements they are making in their eating and body size. Use it as your reference manual.

We have designed the format of this book and our other books in **The Joy of Living Series** to be as simple and direct as possible. You will not have to fish through unnecessary anecdotes and lengthy explanations to get to the information that will help you begin changing your weight and life, now.

Form Your Own Support Group

The best way to have long-term success changing from an overeater to a normal eater is to provide yourself with support along the way. (See p. 301.)

You Have to Be Fed Up with Diets

If you are someone who is not yet utterly dissatisfied and finished with dieting and diet programs, this book may not be right for you. If you still believe that diets might work, as you are reading this book you will probably say to yourself, "I'll try this technique, and if it doesn't work, then I'll go on a diet again." This "diet-around-the-corner" attitude will make you begin planning a diet even as you begin reading, and will almost surely guarantee failure with this technique. This book teaches you how to become your ideal body size by eating whatever you want, not by restricting what you want to eat.

As you will learn in here, and probably know from your own experience, virtually all diets produce binges. If you are mentally preparing for a diet because you are afraid this technique will not work for you, you will most likely use this approach to binge. You will abuse your new freedom that lets you eat whatever you want as the opportunity to advance-binge for the restrictive diet you already may be mentally preparing for.

In other words, if you have not experienced the repeated and total failure of diets and diet programs to produce permanent weight loss, then you still believe that if only you found the right diet that you could stick to, your life-long weight problem would magically go away. If this is the case, then you are hooked on diets, and our diet-free, permanent weight-loss strategy is not for you.

The material in this book has utterly changed the quality of our own lives and the lives of many others by providing permanent freedom from excess weight and overeating. It is our heartfelt wish that it can help you as much as it has helped us.

Who Has Succeeded Using *The Seven Secrets of Slim People*?

- Anyone who regularly struggles with losing the last ten or so pounds.

- People who repeatedly cycle between overeating and restricting food.
- People who eat to alleviate emotions such as stress, sadness, anger, anxiety, loss, etc.
- Compulsive overeaters.
- People who exercise obsessively.
- Health-conscious people who are exasperated by ever-contradictory nutritional and medical information and want clear, accurate, lasting information about how to eat best.
- Mothers with children who want their children to be their natural weight and to be normal, healthy eaters.
- Adolescents, 12 to 20 years old, who are seeking peer approval and are compelled to match social standards of beauty and fitness.
- Former athletes and performers who, in the past, had to abide by restricted diets and have been unable to become normal eaters.
- Obese people.
- Mates, parents, or intimates of any of the above.

The Joy of Living Series

We are dedicated to providing you, our audience, with wisdom and learning in **The Joy of Living Series** of self-improvement books and materials. The series provides manageable, proven solutions for common life challenges. Its format is short, direct, conversational, and supportive. The materials provide truly achievable solutions with measurable results.

The series simply and genuinely enhances the day-to-day meaning and pleasure of central parts of your life. Our titles span Relationships, Money, Life Purpose, Weight and Health, Self-Esteem, and Spirituality.

We derive great strength and knowledge from our audience, and, as always, are grateful for and value your response and contributions. Your voices are the inspiration for our work.

FOR MORE INFORMATION

Call toll-free: (800) 484-2715, code 6750
(The recording directs you to enter code.)

We welcome your call if you would like details on any of the following. (See p. 303.)

1. A free catalog of additional books and tapes in **The Joy of Living Series.**
2. Personal Eating Training—confidential phone consultations.
3. The Seven Secrets of Slim People Support Groups—to join one in your area or begin one.
4. Quantity book purchase discount.
5. Lectures and Workshops.
6. Joy of Living Quarterly Newsletter.

CHAPTER 1

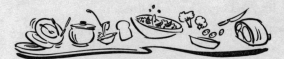

How Does Weight Control Damage You?

American Women and Weight

- The average American woman is 5'4", weighs 140 lbs., and wears a size 14 dress.

- The "ideal" woman, portrayed by models and actresses, is 5'9", and weighs 110 lbs.

- One-third of all American women wear a size 16 or larger.

- 75% of American women are dissatisfied with their appearance.

- 50% of American women are on a diet at any one time.

- Between 90 and 99% of reducing diets fail to produce permanent weight loss.

- Two-thirds of dieters regain the weight within one year. Virtually all regain it within five years.

- Quick weight-loss schemes are among the most common consumer frauds, and diet programs have the highest customer dissatisfaction of any service industry.

- The diet industry takes in over $40 billion each year, and is still growing.

- By contrast, the whole American food industry spends $36 billion annually to advertise its products.[1]

75% of all Americans are overweight, and 33% are obese.[2]

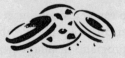

American Girls and Weight

- Young girls are more afraid of becoming fat than they are of nuclear war, cancer, or of losing their parents.

- 50% of 9-year-old girls and 80% of 10-year-old girls have dieted.

- 90% of high school junior and senior women diet regularly, even though only between 10 and 15% are over the weight recommended by the standard height-weight charts.

- 1% of teenage girls and 5% of college-age women become anorexic or bulimic.

- Anorexia has the highest death rate (up to 20%) of any psychiatric diagnosis.

- Girls develop eating and self-image problems before drug or alcohol problems; there are drug and alcohol programs in almost every school, but no eating-disorder programs.[3]

36"-18"-33"

Projected measurements of a Barbie doll if she were a full-sized human being.

33"-23"-33"

Average measurements of a contemporary fashion model.[4]

It's Not Your Fault—You Are Not Alone

- Do you feel personally to blame that you don't have your weight "under control"?

- You are not to blame.

- You were born with a body that knew how to eat perfectly.

- You were *taught* not to listen to your body and therefore not to trust it. This created a "weight" problem.

- 75 to 80% of American women diet and hate their bodies. If this happened to most of the women you've known, what made you think you'd escape?

- Little boys in America are taught to shape their *lives;* little girls are taught to shape their *bodies.*

The cultural message for American women:
Slim = Beauty = Success

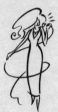

The cultural message for American men:
Effort = Achievement = Success

CHAPTER 2

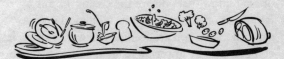

Dieting Has Made You Fatter!

Why Diets Fail

- A diet creates an artificial famine. Your body doesn't know that you are the creator of this famine. It only knows that its biological goal is survival. Since you are feeding it fewer calories, it compensates by lowering its metabolism as much as 40%.[5]

- You may have normally burned 2,000 calories a day. If you only allow yourself 1,200 calories a day for a while, your body will start reducing the number of calories it burns to keep you alive.

- If your metabolism drops by 40%, it will only take 1,200 calories to maintain your *original weight*, and far fewer to maintain a lower weight. So you eat less and less, and can't lose weight permanently.

- If you go back to the 2,000 calories you used to eat, 800 will be stored as fat until your body adjusts to the fact that there is now more food, and raises your metabolism back up again to match your normal caloric intake. THIS ADJUSTMENT MAY TAKE UP TO A YEAR AFTER ONLY ONE DIET![6]

- People typically gain back the weight lost in a diet, PLUS ABOUT 10% more for each diet.[7] But diets fail because you go off of them and ultimately gain *more* weight.

You must feed your body, not starve it, to achieve your ideal weight.

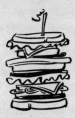

Why Do Diets Make You Fatter?

- You are PHYSIOlogically deprived. Your body is afraid there isn't enough food around to biologically survive, so it wants to OVEREAT when given a chance.

- You are PSYCHOlogically deprived. While on the diet, you did not allow yourself to have what you WANTED.

- So when you "go off your diet," YOU GO CRAZY!

- You say to yourself:

  "I've blown it already. I might as well binge."

  "I'll start over again tomorrow, so I better eat it all now and get it out of the house."

  "I'll definitely start dieting on Monday, so this is my last chance to eat whatever I want."

- The problem is: DEPRIVATION and CONTROL of food CREATE overeating!

- Deprivation and control of food also create an OBSESSION with food.

- Pretty soon, all you can think about is eating.

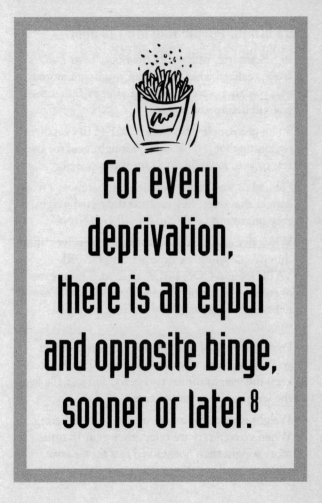

For every deprivation, there is an equal and opposite binge, sooner or later.[8]

Diets Are for People Who Are Too Slim

- Bob Schwartz, who wrote the book, *Diets Don't Work*, realized what the rest of you have ignored—that you always weigh MORE after each diet than you did before you began.

- So he put people who were TOO THIN on diets, reasoning that if diets created weight gain for the rest of you, it would do so for them as well.

- He had to warn these people that there was a real danger that once they reached their goal weight, they might not be able to STOP GAINING.

- Why? Because for the first time in their lives, these thin people would be experiencing DEPRIVATION and CONTROL of food. This creates overeating and food obsession, which would not necessarily stop once they reached their goal weight.

- Diets fail 98% of the time for *everyone* (not just you!). Research indicates that only 10% of dieters keep the weight off for two years, and just 2% keep the weight off for seven years.[9]

- Weight is gained much more easily after dieting. When starved rats are refed, they gain 18 times more weight than nonstarved rats *fed the same amount!*[10]

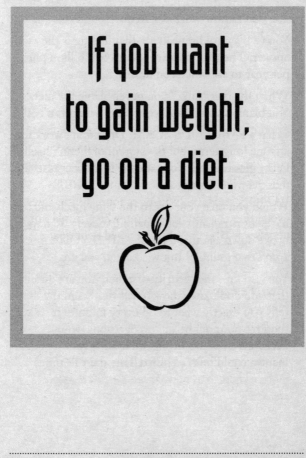

If you want to gain weight, go on a diet.

If It Doesn't Work, Why Do You Keep Dieting?

- You don't know what else to do.

- You've been told repeatedly that dieting is the answer. The diet industry spends $40 billion plus per year to convince you of this.

- When the diet "fails," you never blame the diet. You blame yourself and your "low willpower."

- What a FABULOUS SCAM! Diets don't work for anyone long term, but the system of dieting itself never gets blamed. You take the blame because "it worked while I stuck to it."

- Would you take your car to the same mechanic to have your transmission repaired, if every 30 days it broke down again and he BLAMED YOU? You aren't that gullible! But with diets, you are.

- You also love the security of a diet. You are afraid that you don't know how to eat right, and the diet tells you exactly what to do every minute. It requires no thought and no decisions (your decisions could be wrong, after all!). Your mantra could be . . . "Just tell me the rules."

Your mantra could be . . .

"Just tell me the rules."

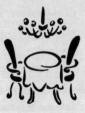

Which Came First, Fat or Thin?

- Thirty years ago, our standard of beauty was the voluptuous size-12 Marilyn Monroe. Today it is the size-2 likes of *Lois and Clark* TV star Teri Hatcher.[11]

- Since only one woman in 40,000 has our currently idealized, model-thin body, it's no wonder that "research shows that virtually all women are ashamed of their bodies today," compared to 23% in 1972.[12]

- Since 1979, Miss America contestants have become so skinny that the majority now are at least 15% below the recommended body weight for their height. (This is a symptom of anorexia nervosa.)[13]

- "Society's standard of beauty is an image that is literally just short of starvation for most women."[14]

- The increase in overweight people in the U.S. parallels the increase in the diet industry. As we discussed before, diets create weight gain.[15]

- The more we, as a nation, have become obsessed with thinness, the fatter we have become.

We are the fattest
industrialized nation
in the world,
yet we are the most
obsessed with thinness.

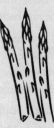

One Diet Can Create an Eating Disorder

- In the 1940s, the University of Minnesota conducted research on the effects of starvation. A group of normal weight and psychologically healthy men were put on a diet that cut their daily intake in half.

- Over 6 months, their average body weight dropped by 25% (which is anorexic).

- Their average basal metabolic rate dropped by 40%.

- After the diet, on the average, it took 14 months of refeeding for their metabolism and weight to return to normal.

- Every single one of these men became either anorexic, bulimic, or an overeater.

- First, they regained the lost weight, plus about 10%. They regained fat first. Eventually, their weight normalized and their percentage of body fat dropped back to their pre-diet levels.

- You, on the other hand, would panic if you gained the lost weight plus 10% and would begin another diet long before the 14 months of refeeding had passed.[16]

Every single one of the men became either anorexic, bulimic, or an overeater.

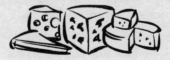

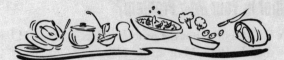

CHAPTER 3

Weight Is Not Your Problem

What Is Your *Real* Problem?

- WEIGHT is not the problem. Excess WEIGHT is the SYMPTOM of the problem.

- If weight were the problem, all you would have to do would be to lose weight successfully one time, and the problem would be solved.

- You have lost weight before and yet it has returned. WHY?

- Because the REAL PROBLEM is OVEREATING. You MUST be putting more food into your body than your body wants. No matter how little YOU THINK you are eating, if you have excess weight, you are OVEReating.*

- But the REAL, REAL PROBLEM is whatever CAUSES the overeating. Let's call it factor "X."

- If you can resolve what CAUSES the overeating, you will stop the overeating and be unable to maintain excess weight.

* (Assuming you have no genetic or metabolic abnormalities.)

Problem
↓
Symptom
↓
Symptom

Factor X
↓
Overeating
↓
Weight

How Can You Pick the *Right* Solution?

- For example, let's say you get a headache every time you go to work. Is the headache THE PROBLEM? No. It is the SYMPTOM of the problem.

- You determine that STRESS is causing the headache. Is STRESS the problem? No. Stress is caused by the real problem, and only you can figure out what that is.

- If it is your BOSS that is causing you STRESS because of excessive daily demands, you will have a headache EVERY DAY unless you address the REAL PROBLEM.

- What you usually do is avoid THE PROBLEM and try to address the SYMPTOMS. For example:

  1. *Take aspirin for the headache.*

  2. *Take a stress-reduction class.*

  3. *Take up meditation.*

  4. *Take up jogging.*

- In this instance, CORRECT problem solving may be:

  1. *Find a new job.*

  2. *Take assertiveness classes to learn boundary setting with your boss.*

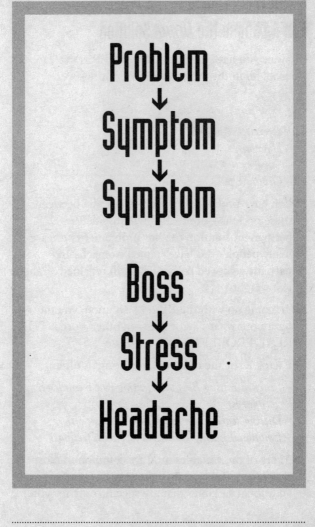

Problem
↓
Symptom
↓
Symptom

Boss
↓
Stress
↓
Headache

If You Think Weight is the *Problem,* You'll Choose the *Wrong* Solution

- Since you have identified WEIGHT as the problem in the past, the known options were:

  – *Diets*
  – *Diet Pills*
  – *Exercise*
  – *Hypnosis*
  – *Surgery*
  – *Giving Up*

- You have probably bounced repeatedly between these options—none of which provided a permanent solution to your problem. (There are many people who have stapled stomachs and partially removed colons who still regained all their lost weight.)

- To come up with the RIGHT solution, you must figure out what Factor X is—in other words, THE REAL PROBLEM.

- Factor X, or the cause of overeating, is often:

  – *Learned Eating Behavior (eating by parental/societal standards)*
  – *Dieting (eating resulting from deprivation)*
  – *Emotional Eating (eating to cope with feelings)*

- Many of the variables in X are common to most overeaters. (Of course, there may be some additional variables that are specific only for you.)

Overeating is often caused by:

- Learned eating behaviors
- Dieting
- Emotional eating

You're Not Crazy; You're Only Making Yourself Crazy

- If a solution repeatedly doesn't work, TRY ITS OPPOSITE!

- What is the opposite behavior of what you have been doing with food?

NOW	OPPOSITE
Overriding your body	→ Trusting your body
Controlling your body	→ Listening to your body
Hating your body	→ Accepting your body
Eating to cope	→ Trusting your feelings
Perfectionism	→ Accepting yourself
Mistrusting yourself	→ Trusting yourself

- You've tried all the rest—give this a test.

- What do you have to lose but weight, despair, and your obsession?

Old Chinese definition of insanity:

"Doing the same thing over and over again and expecting it to turn out differently."

Hating Your Body Doesn't Make It Slimmer

- If hating your body helped, you'd already be as slim as you ever wished to be!

- Hating your body is expressed in many ways.

- For example:
  - *Getting on the scales.*
  - *Keeping clothes that are too small in your closet.*
  - *Looking in the mirror with judgment.*
  - *Wearing clothes that are too tight.*
  - *Not buying new clothes until you are slimmer.*
  - *Not spending money on a great haircut, manicure, pedicure, until you are slimmer.*
  - *Looking at the size labels in clothes.*

- Every one of the above causes *overeating*, not normal eating.

Hating your body only causes you to overeat from shame, self-disgust, and despair.

What Is the Answer?

- If what is causing your overeating is CONTROLLING and MISTRUSTING your body and yourself, then the cure has to be regaining body trust and self-trust.

- We say REGAINING, rather than learning, because you were *born* trusting your body, your feelings, and yourself.

- All of the mistrust and control of your body's physical signals is a LEARNED behavior.

  - *You LEARNED to eat for reasons other than body hunger.*

  - *You LEARNED to diet and to control food.*

  - *You LEARNED to eat in order to cope with feelings.*

  - *You LEARNED to criticize and judge yourself, seeking self-improvement, to make yourself more lovable.*

THE ANSWER IS:

Recovering your natural relationship with food and eating.

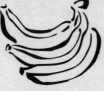

The Seven Secrets of Slim People

1. Listen to Your *Body*, Not Your *Mind*.

2. Eat With *Awareness* and Without *Judgment*.

3. Eat Only When You Are *Physically* Hungry.

4. Stop Eating When You Are *Satisfied*, Not Full.

5. Eat What You Want Most.

6. Notice How Your Body Feels *After* Eating.

7. *Honor* Your Feelings; Don't Bury Them Under Food.

The Seven Secrets of "Naturally" Slim People

CHAPTER 4

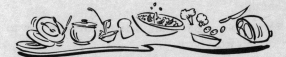

SECRET 1:
Listen to Your *Body,* Not Your *Mind*

Perfect Eating

- PERFECT EATING = Eating in a way that produces your ideal weight and best possible health.

- Your body is genetically designed to know how to do this from birth.

- Have you ever tried to feed a crying baby that you thought was hungry, but was actually wet or tired? Didn't the baby refuse to eat?

- All infants REFUSE to eat except when they are PHYSICALLY HUNGRY. (You did this, too!)

- Once you understood language, your parents taught you to IGNORE or OVERRIDE your body's guidance regarding eating. Instead of letting you eat only when you were hungry, they taught you to eat for many reasons other than physical hunger.

- Your body is a perfect health, weight, and nutrition regulator *FOR YOU!* Your body has never stopped sending you physical messages about how to eat; you just learned to stop listening.

- How your body wants to eat may be very different from how other people's bodies want to eat.

- There is no single answer about how to eat that is right for everyone other than: "Listen to your own body." And luckily for you, the body speaks very clearly, as you will see.

Your body already knows how to eat perfectly.

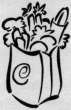

Imperfect Eating

- IMPERFECT EATING = Trusting your mind, or ANY OUTSIDE AUTHORITY (i.e., parents, diets, weight-loss programs, nutrition experts, and doctors), over your own body.

- Your mind is full of messages you LEARNED that told you it was better to trust what your parents told you to do with food, rather than what your body told you to do.

- FOR EXAMPLE:
  - *"Clean your plate."*
  - *"Get your money's worth."*
  - *"A good breakfast is the most important meal of the day."*
  - *"You can't have dessert until you eat your vegetables."*
  - *"Don't eat now; you'll ruin your dinner."*
  - *"If you served it, you eat it."*
  - *"I don't care if you're not hungry; we eat together as a family."*
  - *"Eat this, you'll feel better."*
  - *"If you're good, you can eat ice cream."*

- What messages did you get about eating in your family when you were growing up?

- If you obeyed any of these messages, you were learning to IGNORE or OVERRIDE what your body was telling you to do with food.

Trust your body, not your mind.[17]

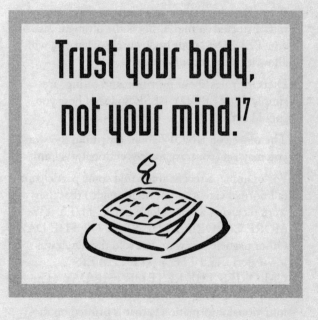

Distorted Eating

- DISTORTED EATING = Not just OVERRIDING or ignoring body signals, but going one step further by attempting to CONTROL your body and TELL IT how to eat.

- If you have ever gone on a diet, you have moved into distorted eating. A diet is the ultimate case of you TELLING your body exactly what you will allow it to eat and when.

- Diets, or rules about nutrition and eating, are simply SOMEBODY ELSE'S idea of how you should eat.

- The more you KNOW about nutrition, the worse you may eat (contrary to conventional wisdom).

- For example, a recent study told some participants (all normal eaters and normal weight) that they were receiving a low-calorie lunch. THEY ATE MORE CALORIES THE REST OF THE DAY. Other participants were not told the lunch was low-calorie, and THEY ATE FEWER CALORIES THE REST OF THE DAY. (The study was seeking to analyze how useful all the nutritional information is that is printed on most food items.)[18]

- By contrast, if dieters drink a high-calorie milkshake, they will eat more the rest of the day, whereas non-dieters will eat less. The dieters say, "I've already blown it, so what's the use?"[19]

If you have a distorted body, the culprit is distorted eating.

What Is a "Naturally" Slim or "Normal" Eater?

- Normal eaters seem to be able to eat regular meals.

- Normal eaters do not obsess about food.

- Normal eaters may overeat occasionally, but do not get upset with themselves about it.

- Normal eaters don't seem to worry about their weight or body.

- Normal eaters don't count calories or fat grams.

- Normal eaters eat a wide variety of foods, even junk food.

- Normal eaters have dessert without guilt.

- We often call normal eaters, "naturally" slim people.

- You probably remember being a normal eater as a child or through your teens. You didn't worry about food or your weight then. You can return to that state. Your body was designed to relate to food normally.

You were born a naturally slim or normal eater.

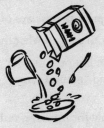

Who Are Naturally Slim People?

- They trust their bodies, not their minds, when it comes to food.

- The only difference between you and naturally slim people is that they refused to accept the parental and societal messages about how they should eat, whereas at some point, you did accept those messages.

- They eat only according to body signals of hunger. They rarely eat for emotional reasons.

- They feel *entitled* to eat whatever they want in front of anyone.

- They *never* deprive themselves of food they want.

- They *never* try to control what they are eating.

- They could not last on a diet for one day because "willpower" and "natural eating" contradict each other.

- They eat mainly for pleasure, rather than to fuel themselves.

- They never judge themselves, no matter what they do with food—including overeating.

Natvally slim people seem to be able to eat whatever they want, whenever they want, and not gain weight.

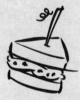

How Do the Naturally Slim Eat?

- They eat only when they are *physically* hungry.

- They eat what they *want most*.

- They stop when their bodies are *satisfied* (comfortable or not hungry anymore) rather than when they are full.

- They give their food their conscious attention when they eat.

- They notice how their bodies feel during and *after* eating.

- They have no "good" or "bad" foods. All foods are to be enjoyed.

- They don't stuff uncomfortable feelings under food.

You were born a naturally slim eater.

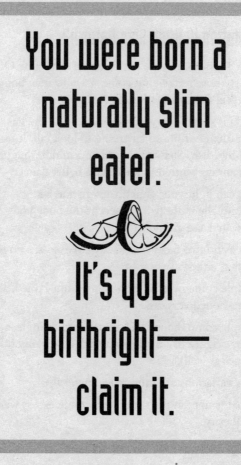

It's your birthright— claim it.

Is Variation in Body Size Natural?

- Can a giraffe reshape itself into an elephant? Of course not. Yet when it comes to your own body, you feel responsible for reshaping it.

- Vikki is short, curvy, and brunette, and she has spent half her life so far trying to look tall, lean, and Swedish. Shawn is built like a middleweight and always wanted to look like a ballet dancer.

- You can fight your genetic design and be continually in despair, or accept the body you inherited and enjoy it.

- Just as no two faces are exactly alike, so are no two bodies, either.

- People come in small-boned, medium-boned, and large-boned versions.

- People come shaped like an inverted triangle, a pear, a figure 8, a circle, or a stick (and many other shapes as well).

- The variations are infinite and *natural*.

- What is not natural is uncomfortable excess weight or obesity.

Ideal bodies come in all shapes and sizes . . .

except fat.

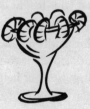

Why Don't You Try to Become Taller or Shorter?

- Because you can't!

- Height is genetically predetermined (although it can be stunted by malnutrition, drugs, etc.) just like eye color and hair color.

- Of course you can alter your eye color with contact lenses and your hair color with dye.

- But no plastic surgeon yet has come up with a way to make you taller or shorter.

- So no matter what your height is, you more or less have had to accept it, right?

- Sure, you can wear platforms and high heels if you're too short, or slouch if you're too tall, but you can't *really* disguise your height from anyone.

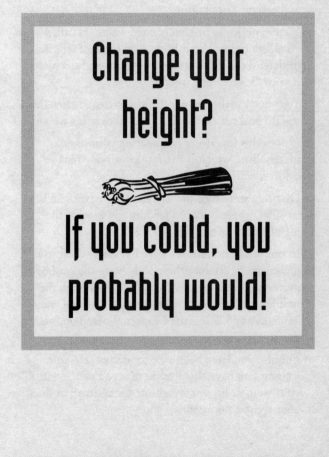

Change your height?

If you could, you probably would!

Is Weight as Impossible to Control as Height?

- Your body was born with a genetically predetermined bone structure, ideal weight, and weight distribution.

- Your genetically predetermined weight is called your "set point." Your body goes to great lengths to defend this genetically designed weight, which is your "ideal" body weight.

- Your body makes it very difficult to lose below this weight and very difficult to gain above this weight.

- It does this by raising or lowering your basal metabolism, which is the rate your body burns calories while at rest.[20]

- Dieting can reduce the metabolic rate from 15% to 40%, whereas forced feeding can *increase* the metabolic rate as much as 75%.

- In one study, volunteers were fed *double* their usual intake over a six-month period—with the goal of increasing their weight 20 to 25%. Although the first few pounds were gained easily, the total weight gained was 75% less than expected based on intake, due to metabolic speed-up.[21]

- Because you have been able to temporarily lose weight, you have the illusion that you can "control" your weight. Is your weight under control, or does your weight now control you?

Changing your genetic weight permanently is as impossible as changing your genetic height.

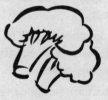

Why Is Obesity Nonexistent in the Wild?

- When a lion kills a gazelle, it doesn't eat the whole animal. Why not?

- The lion eats until it is *satisfied*, not FULL. If it ate to *fullness*, it would get fat and not be able to catch its next meal.

- No matter how much food is available, a wild animal doesn't overeat, even though it cannot put the leftovers in the refrigerator or heat them up in the microwave, as you can.

- You, on the other hand, are never more than five minutes from food, yet you eat like you will never get to eat again.

- A wild animal does not CONTROL its eating. It does what is pleasurable—i.e., eating when hungry, stopping when comfortable.

- Domestic animals can become overweight when you do to them what has been done to you: train them with food, reward them with food, and control their food supply.

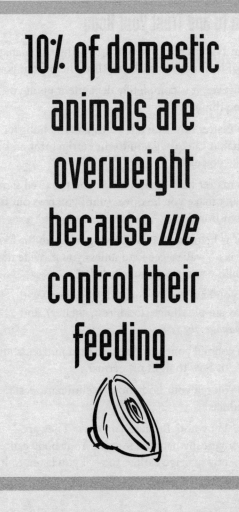

10% of domestic animals are overweight because *we* control their feeding.

Listen to and Trust Your Body

- Your body is completely trustworthy and manages all of its functions with very little help from you.

- However, it is completely dependent upon you for some things.

- No matter how much it sends you the hunger signal, it can't drag you to the refrigerator and make you eat.

- No matter how often it sends you the tired signal, it can't make you lie down (until you pass out from exhaustion).

- It is as helpless as a baby crying in a crib for food. It has no way to get food unless you provide it! Would you starve a hungry baby?

- All you have to do is provide your body with a few simple things (food, rest, shelter), and *it manages the rest.*

- Do you tell your body how to turn nutrients into fuel, or how to fight off germs?

- Do you tell your body how to eliminate waste products?

- No? Why not? Because you *can't!* They are automatically handled for you. Your body can perfectly manage eating, too—if you listen to it!

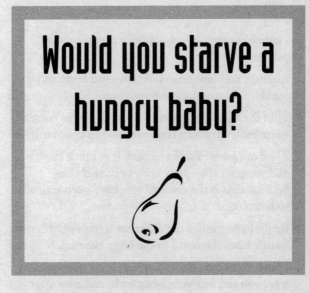

Would you starve a hungry baby?

SECRET 1:
Listen to Your Body, Not Your Mind

WEEK-ONE ASSIGNMENTS

Goals:

1. Gather information about your current eating patterns.

2. Increase your awareness of how your body and mind are communicating with you.

3. Find the right body-signal channel to tune into, a must before you can start listening to your body.

4. Tune out your mind's channel. It is much louder and stronger than your body's channel now, because that is the channel you have been trained to listen to.

5. Begin to recognize the different signals in order to switch from the mind to the body channel.

6. **Daily:** record on the following charts *when* you eat, *what* you eat, *how* your body feels, and *what* your mind says about your choices. Record even if you just had a bite of something. (If you are reluctant to write in this book, please photocopy or duplicate the charts for your own notebook.)

SECRET 1:
Listen to Your *Body*, Not Your *Mind*

example
Body/Mind Awareness Log

Make appropriate comments under each column.

Time	What Food You Ate	How Your Body Felt	What Your Mind Said
6:30AM	3 cups of coffee	Sleepy, sluggish, acid indigestion	You need coffee to get going.
9:00AM	Doughnut/ coffee	Tired, then sugar high, then tired again	Why didn't you eat a healthy breakfast? Here you go again eating sugar.
12:00 noon	Chicken Caesar salad, diet soda	Good	Good, healthy choice, keep it up the rest of the day.
9:00PM	A Whopper with fries and a shake	Starving to stuffed	You pig! You blew it. You didn't need any of that—when will you ever learn?

SECRET 1:
Listen to Your *Body*, Not Your *Mind*

Body/Mind Awareness Log
DAY ONE

Make appropriate comments under each column.

Time	What Food You Ate	How Your Body Felt	What Your Mind Said

SECRET 1:
Listen to Your *Body*, Not Your *Mind*

Body/Mind Awareness Log
DAY TWO

Make appropriate comments under each column.

Time	What Food You Ate	How Your Body Felt	What Your Mind Said

SECRET 1:
Listen to Your *Body*, Not Your *Mind*

Body/Mind Awareness Log
DAY THREE

Make appropriate comments under each column.

Time	What Food You Ate	How Your Body Felt	What Your Mind Said

SECRET 1:
Listen to Your *Body*, Not Your *Mind*

Body/Mind Awareness Log
DAY FOUR

Make appropriate comments under each column.

Time	What Food You Ate	How Your Body Felt	What Your Mind Said

SECRET 1:
Listen to Your *Body*, Not Your *Mind*

Body/Mind Awareness Log
DAY FIVE

Make appropriate comments under each column.

Time	What Food You Ate	How Your Body Felt	What Your Mind Said

SECRET 1:
Listen to Your *Body*, Not Your *Mind*

Body/Mind Awareness Log
DAY SIX

Make appropriate comments under each column.

Time	What Food You Ate	How Your Body Felt	What Your Mind Said

SECRET 1:
Listen to Your *Body*, Not Your *Mind*

Body/Mind Awareness Log
DAY SEVEN

Make appropriate comments under each column.

Time	What Food You Ate	How Your Body Felt	What Your Mind Said

End of Week One—What Did You Learn?

(PLEASE WRITE IN THE BLANKS)

Body

- List the ways your body communicated with you (e.g., hunger, sugar high, stuffed, exhaustion, nervous eating, indigestion, gas).

- What made your body feel good (e.g., kind of food, quantity, time of eating)?

- What made your body feel bad?

- How could you tell the difference between a body message and a mind message?

End of Week One—What Did You Learn?

(PLEASE WRITE IN THE BLANKS)

Mind

• How did your mind communicate with you?

• How helpful or unhelpful were your mind's comments?

• Did you feel supported by your mind, or criticized?

• How many of your mind's messages can you trace to an original outside source?

Additional Notes for the Week

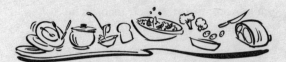

CHAPTER 5

SECRET 2:

Eat With *Awareness*

and Without

Judgment

Become a Scientific Observer of Your Own Body

- Do you remember the scientific method from school? Scientists test their theories by experimenting and observing the outcome.

- *Suspend judgment.* Scientists must remain *objective* or they will influence the outcome through their preconceived beliefs. Try to be a scientific observer of your eating, not a judge. (Suspending judgment may be the most difficult part of becoming a normal eater.)

- You don't need to BELIEVE that your body is trustworthy; you only need to test for yourself whether this theory is true or false: "My body can be completely trusted to tell me how to eat to be my ideal weight and health."

- You can become a complete expert on your own body by simply eating with awareness of how your body feels before, during, and after eating.

- Your body's feedback comes in the form of hunger, fullness, comfort, discomfort, pleasure, tastiness, tastelessness, etc.

- To learn to listen to and trust your body again is going to take some practice. You need to become aware of how the body communicates with you before you can possibly listen to it.

- You cannot become aware while you are criticizing yourself.

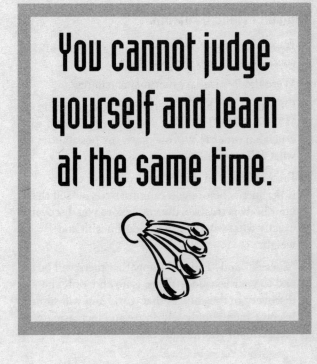

You cannot judge
yourself and learn
at the same time.

You Can't Make a Mistake

- It took Thomas Edison over 1,000 experiments to successfully invent the light bulb.

- Were the 999 initial experiments failures?

- Of course not! Each experiment showed Edison *WHAT DIDN'T WORK*, and that information was crucial in order to narrow down the possibilities of what *DID* work.

- Pretend that you need 1,000 conscious eating experiments before you can prove to yourself that your body is trustworthy and before you discover exactly what works for your ideal health and weight.

- "Success" and "Failure" imply that there will be an end to your learning. There is no end, only the discovery of the choices that work. You will simply become increasingly self-aware and increasingly respectful of your unique body.

There is no success and no failure in learning.

Being Conscious of Your Eating May Feel Odd at First

- Do you remember when you first learned to drive a car? It was difficult to focus your attention on the side view mirrors, the rear view mirrors, the boundaries of the car, the traffic, and signals all at the same time.

- Now, you can probably drive from point A to point B and not remember the drive at all. Driving has become completely unconscious.

- You were designed to have perfect eating be a completely unconscious process. It will become unconscious again, after you learn to trust your body.

- For right now, though, you must become very conscious of this natural eating process, in order to listen to it and test it.

- Just know that before long you will simply relax and eat, just as you relax and breathe.

Ultimately, perfect eating will be as easy and unconscious as breathing.

A Conscious Eating Experiment

- Select an assortment of favorite foods and put a small piece of each on a plate. For example: a potato chip, a pickle slice, a piece of cheese, a raisin, a slice of apple, a piece of salami, etc.

- Ask a friend to do this with you. If not, you can do it on your own. If you are with a friend, shut your eyes and have the friend pick a piece of food and hold it under your nose to smell, and then have him or her feed you.

- When a bite goes in your mouth, keep your eyes closed and suck on it first—move it around in your mouth and notice the different flavors and textures at different locations in your mouth.

- Then chew the food, swallow, and notice the aftertaste. Continue through all of the foods on the plate.

- Did each item taste as you expected? Did you like the smell better than the taste of some foods? Or vice versa? Did you like certain textures more than others? Did you like sucking better than chewing? Did you like the aftertaste? Each bite is a total experience—keep experiencing the totality!

- Do a conscious eating experiment and record your experiment on page 90.

Eating with your eyes closed may make you more aware.

Eat Consciously

- To become more conscious of your eating:

- *Sit down*—even if it is one bite of ice cream—take the spoon and *sit down*. If you taste while you are cooking, go to a chair and *sit down* to taste.

- *Eat without distractions.* For the next six weeks, do not eat and read, eat and watch TV, eat and drive, or eat and do *anything* else at the same time. You cannot become conscious while distracted.

- How would you feel if tonight, while you were sleeping, a cookie monster stuffed 10 lbs. of fresh, homemade chocolate chip cookies into your body, and tomorrow you weighed 10 lbs. more?

- Would you be angry if you weighed 10 lbs. more and didn't get to taste a single bite? Of course you would! Yet anytime you eat and do *anything* else at the same time, the cookie monster is at work!

- When you eat unconsciously, you only deprive yourself of the total pleasure of the food. You get the calories, without the fun.

- Eating is designed to be emotionally as well as physically satisfying. If you watch TV and eat a sandwich, you will have been distracted from enjoying at least half of the sandwich. Your body will have a full sandwich in it, but emotionally you will feel like you only ate a half sandwich because that is all you noticed and enjoyed! That will leave you wanting more.

Unconscious eating unleashes the cookie monster in you.

Disconnect the Eating Machine[22]

- You may tend to eat automatically. Once you get your hands on a fork, the hand-to-mouth action doesn't end until the food is all gone.

- In order to be aware and take more pleasure in your food (*not* to slow you down so you will eat less), put your fork down after each bite and do not pick it up again until your mouth is empty.

- Do the same thing if you are eating a sandwich or a roll. Hands completely *off* of the food while there is a bite in your mouth. When your mouth is *empty*, pick up your food again.

- If you find that putting your utensil down is difficult to remember, try eating with your non-dominant hand. That may be awkward enough to remind you.

- If you are busy organizing your next bite, or have a bite waiting on your fork, you only deprive yourself of the pleasure of the food in your mouth.

You cannot really enjoy the bite in your mouth if another bite is waiting on your fork.

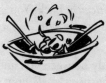

Eat What You Want in Front of Anyone

- You may not feel *entitled* to eat what you want until you are slim. You are afraid people will judge you and say, "No wonder you're fat; look at what you're eating!"

- Lack of entitlement *makes* you fat!

- If no one sees you do it, it didn't really happen. It's a way you hide from yourself and everyone else. You feel forced to eat in secret.

- Normal eaters eat whatever they want in front of anyone. To become a normal eater, you *must* do the same.

- Take your *entitlement* back! You aren't going to give up eating until you're slim. In fact, you *must* eat to become slim.

- Eating is strictly between you and your body. It is no one else's business *at all*, how, what, or when you eat.

- Do you feel *entitled* to go to the bathroom whenever your body says so? It's the *same thing*.

You are *entitled* to eat whatever you want in front of anyone *regardless* of your body size.

SECRET 2:
Eat *With* Awareness and *Without* Judgment

WEEK-TWO ASSIGNMENTS

1. Conduct the conscious eating experiment described on page 82. The date I did this was _____. What I learned from this was:

2. Whenever you eat anything:

   a) Sit down.

   b) Eat consciously and without distractions.

   c) Hands off the food or utensils between bites.

   d) Eat in front of whomever is around.

   e) Observe and record your experiment daily in the body awareness log—check off what you did each time.

SECRET 2:
Eat *With* Awareness and *Without* Judgment

example
Body Awareness Log

Check off what you did each time, and record any appropriate comments.

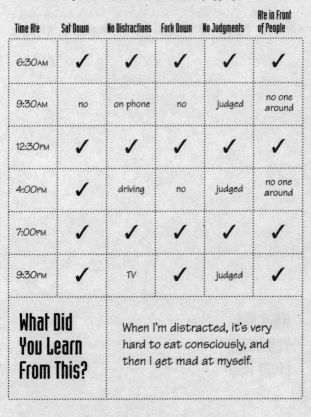

Time Ate	Sat Down	No Distractions	Fork Down	No Judgments	Ate in Front of People
6:30AM	✓	✓	✓	✓	✓
9:30AM	no	on phone	no	judged	no one around
12:30PM	✓	✓	✓	✓	✓
4:00PM	✓	driving	no	judged	no one around
7:00PM	✓	✓	✓	✓	✓
9:30PM	✓	TV	✓	judged	✓

What Did You Learn From This?

When I'm distracted, it's very hard to eat consciously, and then I get mad at myself.

SECRET 2:
Eat *With* Awareness and *Without* Judgment

Body Awareness Log
DAY ONE

Check off what you did each time, and record any appropriate comments.

Time Ate	Sat Down	No Distractions	Fork Down	No Judgments	Ate in Front of People

What Did You Learn From This?

SECRET 2:
Eat *With* Awareness and *Without* Judgment

Body Awareness Log
DAY TWO

Check off what you did each time, and record any appropriate comments.

Time Ate	Sat Down	No Distractions	Fork Down	No Judgments	Ate in Front of People
What Did You Learn From This?					

SECRET 2:
Eat *With* Awareness and *Without* Judgment

Body Awareness Log
DAY THREE

Check off what you did each time, and record any appropriate comments.

Time Ate	Sat Down	No Distractions	Fork Down	No Judgments	Ate in Front of People
What Did You Learn From This?					

SECRET 2:
Eat *With* Awareness and *Without* Judgment

Body Awareness Log
DAY FOUR

Check off what you did each time, and record any appropriate comments.

Time Ate	Sat Down	No Distractions	Fork Down	No Judgments	Ate in Front of People
What Did You Learn From This?					

SECRET 2:
Eat *With* Awareness and *Without* Judgment

Body Awareness Log
DAY FIVE

Check off what you did each time, and record any appropriate comments.

Time Ate	Sat Down	No Distractions	Fork Down	No Judgments	Ate in Front of People
What Did You Learn From This?					

SECRET 2:
Eat *With* Awareness and *Without* Judgment

Body Awareness Log
DAY SIX

Check off what you did each time, and record any appropriate comments.

Time Ate	Sat Down	No Distractions	Fork Down	No Judgments	Ate in Front of People

What Did You Learn From This?

SECRET 2:
Eat *With* Awareness and *Without* Judgment

Body Awareness Log
DAY SEVEN

Check off what you did each time, and record any appropriate comments.

Time Ate	Sat Down	No Distractions	Fork Down	No Judgments	Ate in Front of People

What Did You Learn From This?

Additional Notes for the Week

CHAPTER 6

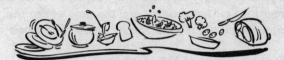

SECRET 3:

Eat Only When You Are *Physically* Hungry

What Does Physical Hunger Feel Like?

Many of you have forgotten what it feels like to be physically hungry. Yet, the only way to be a normal eater is to eat for pleasure, and the only way to really enjoy food is to eat when you are physically hungry.

THIS IS HUNGER! YOU MAY FEEL:

- Empty.
- Lightheaded.
- Slightly nauseated.
- Loss of energy.
- Loss of concentration.
- Irritable, cranky.
- Slight headache.
- Stomachache.
- Hunger pang in stomach.
- Certainty that you *must* eat *now*.

THIS IS NOT HUNGER:

- Salivation just because you saw or smelled food (assuming you weren't feeling hungry before).
- Searching through the cupboards to find something to satisfy a mouth craving (taste).
- The oral urge to chew, chomp, or suck due to anger or anxiety.
- Thirst.
- Stomach tension from nerves.
- Low energy from lack of sleep.
- Sadness, anger, frustration.

When was the last time you were truly hungry?

What did it feel like?

Other Signs of True Hunger

- Anything you eat tastes absolutely wonderful.

- It's impossible for anything to distract you; you can think only about food.

- Usually, some very specific food starts screaming at you in your mind. BEFORE you go into a restaurant, you know EXACTLY what you want. Or something literally jumps out at you from the menu and begs to be ordered.

- Hunger is the best seasoning. If your food is tasteless, or requires extra salt, pepper, ketchup, or Tabasco, you are not hungry.

- If you are hungry, NOTHING interests you more than sitting down and eating and savoring your food. If you feel compelled to do ANYTHING else at the same time you eat, such as watch TV, read, or drive a car, YOU ARE NOT HUNGRY.

- If you say to yourself, "I SHOULD be hungry, I haven't eaten all day," or "I SHOULDN'T be hungry, I just ate," you are not listening to your body. Hunger does not follow a clock or your "shoulds."

- Discomfort isn't hunger. If you are experiencing an uncomfortable feeling, or gas, it is probably that the combination of foods you put in your stomach last time you ate didn't agree with you. Eating more won't make you feel better. To feel better, wait for your body to digest the food.

If you have any *doubts*
about whether you
are hungry or not,
you're not!

True hunger is
unmistakable.

More Hunger Hints

- When you are hungry, even your least favorite food tastes good.

- Hunger is erratic. It comes and goes. If you can't eat when you first get hungry, hunger will disappear for an hour or two and return later. Even though the signal disappears, it still means you *must* eat when it first occurs—*not* ignore it.

- Hunger may come frequently one day, and not at all the next. Trust it.

- Hunger almost never occurs at conventional mealtimes. How inconvenient!

- Preventative eating is not hunger related. It is simply a fear that hunger may show up at an inconvenient time. To prevent possible hunger, we eat what we may need in advance. This is pure body abuse.

- THE MOST VALID REASON TO WAIT UNTIL YOU ARE HUNGRY TO EAT IS BECAUSE THAT'S THE TIME WHEN THE FOOD TASTES THE BEST AND GIVES YOU THE MOST PLEASURE. Your body wants you to experience pleasure, not deprivation or abuse. After you have had enough experiences of how incredible food tastes when you are truly hungry, you will actually begin to relish the prospect of hunger, and insist on waiting for its arrival before you eat!

Hunger may come frequently one day, and not at all the next.

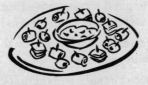

Assess Your Hunger Level

- Imagine that the gas gauge in your car holds *10* gallons. If the indicator is at *10*, your tank is full. If it is at *0*, it is empty.

- You are going to use a similar gauge to help you fine-tune your awareness of your hunger level.

  > *0-Absolutely Starved—you will overeat.*
  > *1-Too Hungry to Care What You Eat— you will overeat.*
  > *2-Seriously Hungry—you must eat now!*
  > *3-Moderately Hungry—could wait longer.*
  > *4-Slightly Hungry—first thoughts of food.*
  > *5-Satisfied, Comfortable—not hungry.*
  > *6-Slightly Uncomfortable—you feel the food.*
  > *7-Uncomfortable—sleepy, sluggish.*
  > *8-Very Uncomfortable—stomach hurts.*
  > *9-Stuffed.*
  > *10-In Pain.*

- If you try to put more gas in your car than 10 gallons, it will run out on the ground.

- If you put more food in your body than it wants, it runs out onto your hips.

- Your stomach's *actual size* is the amount of food it takes to go from a *0* to a *5*. But being biological, it has the ability to *stretch* to a *10* to hold excess, unlike your car.

- Although you want to be truly hungry to eat (at a *2*), you don't want to be TOO hungry. If you are at a *0* or *1*, you *will overeat*.

Your body only wants to eat between a 2 and a 5, hunger and satisfaction.

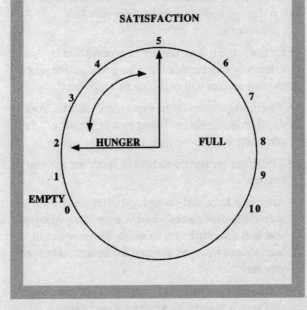

Pleasure Is the Key

- Your body was designed to motivate you to do all the things necessary for your survival by making these things extremely *pleasurable*.

- All animals know when to eat or not, as do people, based on pleasure or pain:

    – *Getting too hungry is painful.*
    – *Eating when hungry is very pleasurable.*
    – *Overeating is painful.*
    – *Stopping at satisfaction is very pleasurable because you feel great, light, and energetic in your body afterwards.*

- By the same token, the act of procreation is extremely pleasurable, because pleasure ensures that all species will continue to reproduce!

- Your body wants you to experience pleasure, not deprivation or abuse. Being in a fit, healthy, attractive body is very pleasurable.

- The more pleasure you find in food, the *less* you'll overeat!

- After you have had enough experiences of how incredible food tastes when you are truly hungry, you will actually begin to relish the prospect of hunger and insist on waiting for its arrival before you eat!

- Focus on the pleasure. If food isn't pleasurable, you're not hungry, or you're eating boring food.

The best reason to wait for hunger is:

That's when food tastes the best!

Eat a Fist Size of Food—
Your Personal Portion Guide

- Make a fist with your hand. Look at it. This is the *approximate* amount of food that your body wants in order to take you from hunger to satisfaction.

- A fist size is also the *approximate* size of your stomach when it is not stretched out. No matter how often you have stretched your stomach, it still sends the signals of satisfaction at *approximately* a fist-size amount of food.

- This is an APPROXIMATE GUIDELINE ONLY! If you are eating consciously, you will find that *usually* a fist size of food is all you want. Sometimes you will want much more; sometimes, only a few bites.

- The portion sizes you are served in restaurants (or even at home) are more appropriate for someone doing hard physical labor 12 hours a day, and have little correlation to your own body's signal for the quantity of food it prefers.

- This DOES NOT MEAN you are limited to a fist size of food at only three meals a day. It DOES mean if you eat a fist size *every time* you get hungry, you will probably get hungry and eat more often.

- Small, frequent amounts of food prevent future binging and also fire up the metabolism. Frequent eating also keeps your blood sugar up so you experience fewer mood and energy swings.

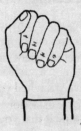

Your body only wants *about* a fist size of food at any one feeding.

Stop Preventative Eating

- Preventative eating is when you eat, although you are not hungry, to prevent hunger from coming later at a *possibly* inconvenient time.

- This is pure body abuse!

- Preventative eating represents a fear of hunger. In order to assure yourself that you always will have food when you are hungry, for now, carry favorite foods with you everywhere. Rather than eat to *prevent* hunger, promise yourself that you can eat some of your stash as soon as you *are* hungry.

- It is tremendously reassuring and secure to know that food is readily available the *moment* you need it.

- Eating preventatively is not pleasurable or satisfying. It is putting food into your body when it *doesn't want it!*

- A good example of this may be eating breakfast even though your *body* isn't hungry until hours later.

- *Any* food that goes into your body when you are not hungry has no place to go except to storage, namely, fat.

You can't eat now to satisfy a hunger yet to come.

Stop Being an "Efficient Eater"

• Under the guise of being "efficient," you eat on the run and eat while you are trying to do other things.

• This is incredibly *inefficient*. If you don't take the *time* to eat now, you will take *much more* time later for diets, gyms, and diet foods to make up for being such an "efficient eater."

• If your entire value is wrapped up in being productive, it's no wonder it's so hard to *only eat* when you eat and do *nothing* else. Since eating only pleasures and benefits you, it seems unproductive!

• How *very* wrong you are! You must feed and nourish yourself before you have the *energy* to produce for everyone else!

• Similar to being "efficient" is being a "neat" eater. That means you feel you have to eat *exactly* half a sandwich—no more, no less—or you have to empty your plate.

• A conscious eater is never neat. Hunger requires either a bite or two more or less than you served yourself. It is *never* neat.

• Stop being efficient and neat with food.

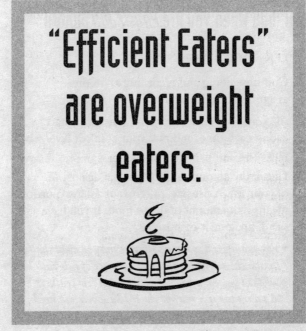

"Efficient Eaters" are overweight eaters.

SECRET 3:
Eat Only When You Are *Physically* Hungry

WEEK-THREE ASSIGNMENTS

1. Continue doing and recording all of the assignments in Week Two.

2. Also, assess your hunger level when you start eating each time, and rate your comfort level when you stop.

3. Check the amount of food you eat against the size of your fist. A fist size, in terms of a dense portion, means that amount of dense food. If you have a salad, imagine it compacted.

   • *For example, a woman's fist size may be about half a sandwich; a large apple; a half a piece of fish with half a baked potato; a bowl of soup with a few crackers, etc. A man's fist size may be closer to a whole sandwich; soup and salad; a whole piece of fish and a small potato; a large apple and a slice of cheese, etc.*

SECRET 3:
Eat Only When You Are *Physically* Hungry

example

Body Awareness Log

Check off what you did. In hunger columns, enter the number that applies.

Time	Sat Down	No Distractions	Fork Down	No Judgment	Hunger Level Start	Comfort Level Stop	Fist Size	Ate in Front of People
7AM	✓	✓	✓	✓	3	6	✓	✓
10AM	no	no	no	no	5	7	✓	✓
2PM	✓	✓	✓	✓	2	5	✓	✓
7PM	✓	✓	✓	✓	5	7	✓	✓
10PM	no	no	no	no	6	7	no	no

What Did You Learn from This?

That I ate <u>before</u> I was hungry in the morning for fear I'd get hungry later. That it's easier for me to wait for hunger at lunchtime than anytime afterwards.

SECRET 3:
Eat Only When You Are *Physically* Hungry

Body Awareness Log
DAY ONE

Check off what you did. In hunger columns, enter the number that applies.

Time	Sat Down	No Distractions	Fork Down	No Judgment	Hunger Level Start	Comfort Level Stop	Fist Size	Ate in Front of People

What Did You Learn from This?

SECRET 3:
Eat Only When You Are *Physically* Hungry

Body Awareness Log
DAY TWO

Check off what you did. In hunger columns, enter the number that applies.

Time	Sat Down	No Distractions	Fork Down	No Judgment	Hunger Level Start	Comfort Level Stop	Fist Size	Ate in Front of People

What Did You Learn from This?

SECRET 3:
Eat Only When You Are *Physically* Hungry

Body Awareness Log
DAY THREE

Check off what you did. In hunger columns, enter the number that applies.

Time	Sat Down	No Distractions	Fork Down	No Judgment	Hunger Level Start	Comfort Level Stop	Fist Size	Ate in Front of People

What Did You Learn from This?

SECRET 3:
Eat Only When You Are *Physically* Hungry

Body Awareness Log
DAY FOUR

Check off what you did. In hunger columns, enter the number that applies.

Time	Sat Down	No Distractions	Fork Down	No Judgment	Hunger Level Start	Comfort Level Stop	Fist Size	Ate in Front of People

What Did You Learn from This?

SECRET 3:
Eat Only When You Are *Physically* Hungry

Body Awareness Log
DAY FIVE

Check off what you did. In hunger columns, enter the number that applies.

Time	Sat Down	No Distractions	Fork Down	No Judgment	Hunger Level Start	Comfort Level Stop	Fist Size	Ate in Front of People

What Did You Learn from This?

SECRET 3:
Eat Only When You Are *Physically* Hungry

Body Awareness Log
DAY SIX

Check off what you did. In hunger columns, enter the number that applies.

Time	Sat Down	No Distractions	Fork Down	No Judgment	Hunger Level Start	Comfort Level Stop	Fist Size	Ate in Front of People

What Did You Learn from This?

SECRET 3:
Eat Only When You Are *Physically* Hungry

Body Awareness Log
DAY SEVEN

Check off what you did. In hunger columns, enter the number that applies.

Time	Sat Down	No Distractions	Fork Down	No Judgment	Hunger Level Start	Comfort Level Stop	Fist Size	Ate in Front of People

What Did You Learn from This?

Additional Notes for the Week

CHAPTER 7

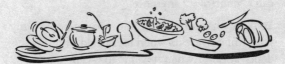

SECRET 4:

Stop Eating When You Are *Satisfied,* Not *Full*

When Does Your Body Want to Stop Eating?

- You may think that your *body* is the culprit and has betrayed you into overeating, when you feel you can't "control it" anymore.

- Your *body* has no interest in overeating *ever*. Only your mind overeats when it is afraid of future deprivation or when it wants to escape uneasy feelings.

- Your *body* wants to stop at satisfaction (at a 5). Satisfaction is when you:

  – *Are not hungry anymore; you feel comfortable.*

  – *Don't* feel *the food in your body.*

  – *Feel light and energetic after eating.*

  – Could *eat more, but you could also wait.*

  – *Find the flavor of the food begins to fade; it goes from* fabulous *to cardboard or sand.*

  – *Are eating, and it becomes harder to give every bite your total attention.*

- Satisfaction is physical AND emotional. Eat emotionally comforting foods when you want them, but only when you are hungry.

- If you eat what you want most *first*, you will become *satisfied* the fastest, and consume the fewest amount of calories.

If you don't wait for the signal to start (hunger),

you'll never hear the signal to stop (satisfaction).

THEY ARE LINKED!

Your Body Never Wants to Be Full

- There are degrees of fullness or discomfort, but they are all *past* the point where your body wants to stop eating.

- Too full is:
  - *Any feeling of the food in your body.*
  - *Loosening your belt.*
  - *Pressing your chest or stomach due to acidic feeling.*
  - *Feeling sluggish or sleepy.*
  - *Feeling uncomfortable.*
  - *Painful.*
  - *Feeling lazy or tired.*
  - *Feeling stuffed.*
  - *Feeling drugged.*
  - *When clothing feels tighter than when you started eating.*

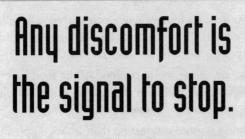

Any discomfort is the signal to stop.

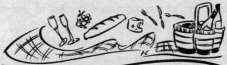

When You Find it Hard to Stop at Satisfaction

If you find it hard to stop at satisfaction, then:

- You didn't *wait* for hunger before you began eating. It's very hard to recognize satisfaction, (at a *5*) if you start at slightly hungry, (at a *4*)!
  Solution? Wait for hunger.

- You were *too* hungry when you started eating. If you eat at a *1* or *0*, you *will overeat* (and so would anyone). *Solution? You must eat at a 2.*

- You are eating mediocre food. If the food isn't *fabulous*, you will keep eating and eating, searching for satisfaction. *Solution? Eat only great food.*

- Eating is more interesting than what you plan to do next. So, of course, you will want to *prolong* the eating to avoid the next uninteresting thing. *Solution? Follow eating with something equally as interesting* (e.g., read a novel, watch a movie, have sex, etc.).

- You are suppressing an emotional hunger. *Solution? Find a better match.* A doughnut will never take the place of a hug when a hug is what you really need.

- When you don't have enough of a particular food in your life. *Solution? Have it more often, not less.*

There is *never* a legitimate reason to eat when you are not hungry or to eat past satisfaction.[23]

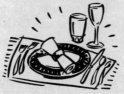

Resign From the "Clean-Your-Plate" Club

- We never understood how cleaning our plates was going to help the starving children in China, but we internalized our parents' messages, nonetheless.

- If you're like us, your parents survived the Depression, and it became important to them not to waste food. They passed that on to you.

- Americans, in general, glorify abundance. Perhaps it comes from the struggles of our predecessors. We have the biggest and best-stocked super-markets in the world.

- One of the ways you decide if a restaurant is great is based on portion size. If you are given a lot of food for your money, *that means good value.*

- The French think we're nuts. The more expensive the French restaurant, the *smaller* the portion size. They believe great dining is about *quality*, not *quantity.*

- You are served portion sizes in restaurants that are more suited to a manual laborer. *What someone else serves you is not your portion size!*

- Taste everything; finish nothing.

Taste everything; finish nothing.[24]

Get Your "Money's Worth" by Increasing Your Awareness of the Total Experience

It's time to rethink what constitutes value for your money when you go out to eat.

Only a small part of what you are paying for goes toward food. Most of your restaurant dollar goes toward:

- Ambiance and decor (music, flowers, candles, etc.).
- Someone to buy the food.
- Someone to cook the food.
- Someone to wait on you and serve it.
- Someone to do the dishes.
- Rent, utilities.
- Laundry service (linen and napkins).
- Inventory (e.g., wine storage).
- Credit card charges.
- And the list goes on.

Consider that you are not paying for the *food*, but that you are paying for the *total experience* of being pampered and catered to. You are paying "booth rent"!

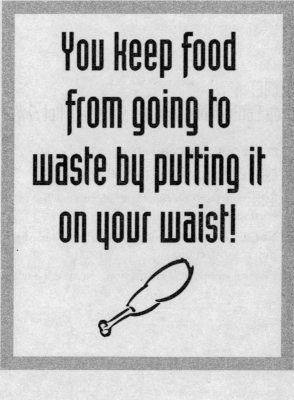

You keep food from going to waste by putting it on your waist!

SECRET 4:
Stop Eating When You Are *Satisfied*, Not *Full*

WEEK-FOUR ASSIGNMENTS

1. Continue keeping your Body Awareness Log.

2. Especially focus on *noticing* when you reach satisfaction.

3. Notice what your mind tells you when it's hard to stop at satisfaction.

4. Practice stopping at satisfaction, one time a day.

SECRET 4:
Stop Eating When You Are *Satisfied*, Not *Full*

example

Body Awareness Log

Check off what you did. In hunger columns, enter the number that applies.

Time	Sat Down	No Distractions	Fork Down	No Judgment	Hunger Level Start	Comfort Level Stop	Fist Size	What Your Mind Said About Stopping
7:30AM	✓	no	✓	✓	3	6	✓	I always read the paper with breakfast.
12:30PM	✓	no	✓	✓	2	7	no	It won't taste as good later.
6:00PM	✓	no	✓	✓	2	6	✓	Don't waste food
9:00PM	✓	no	✓	✓	5	7	no	I deserve a reward—I had a hard day.

What Did You Learn from This?

The hardest thing for me is to eat without distractions. I always read while I eat. I realize being distracted made it hard to recognize my satisfaction signal.

SECRET 4:
Stop Eating When You Are *Satisfied*, Not *Full*

Body Awareness Log
DAY ONE

Check off what you did. In hunger columns, enter the number that applies.

Time	Sat Down	No Distractions	Fork Down	No Judgment	Hunger Level Start	Comfort Level Stop	Fist Size	What Your Mind Said About Stopping

What Did You Learn from This?

SECRET 4:
Stop Eating When You Are *Satisfied*, Not *Full*

Body Awareness Log
DAY TWO

Check off what you did. In hunger columns, enter the number that applies.

Time	Sat Down	No Distractions	Fork Down	No Judgment	Hunger Level Start	Comfort Level Stop	Fist Size	What Your Mind Said About Stopping

What Did You Learn from This?

SECRET 4:
Stop Eating When You Are *Satisfied*, Not *Full*

Body Awareness Log
DAY THREE

Check off what you did. In hunger columns, enter the number that applies.

Time	Sat Down	No Distractions	Fork Down	No Judgment	Hunger Level Start	Comfort Level Stop	Fist Size	What Your Mind Said About Stopping

What Did You Learn from This?

SECRET 4:
Stop Eating When You Are *Satisfied*, Not *Full*

Body Awareness Log
DAY FOUR

Check off what you did. In hunger columns, enter the number that applies.

Time	Sat Down	No Distractions	Fork Down	No Judgment	Hunger Level Start	Comfort Level Stop	Fist Size	What Your Mind Said About Stopping

What Did You Learn from This?

SECRET 4:
Stop Eating When You Are *Satisfied*, Not *Full*

Body Awareness Log
DAY FIVE

Check off what you did. In hunger columns, enter the number that applies.

Time	Sat Down	No Distractions	Fork Down	No Judgment	Hunger Level Start	Comfort Level Stop	Fist Size	What Your Mind Said About Stopping

What Did You Learn from This?

SECRET 4:
Stop Eating When You Are *Satisfied*, Not *Full*

Body Awareness Log
DAY SIX

Check off what you did. In hunger columns, enter the number that applies.

Time	Sat Down	No Distractions	Fork Down	No Judgment	Hunger Level Start	Comfort Level Stop	Fist Size	What Your Mind Said About Stopping

What Did You Learn from This?

SECRET 4:
Stop Eating When You Are *Satisfied*, Not *Full*

Body Awareness Log
DAY SEVEN

Check off what you did. In hunger columns, enter the number that applies.

Time	Sat Down	No Distractions	Fork Down	No Judgment	Hunger Level Start	Comfort Level Stop	Fist Size	What Your Mind Said About Stopping

What Did You Learn from This?

Additional Notes for the Week

CHAPTER 8

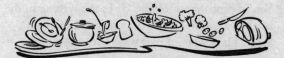

SECRET 5:
Eat What You
Want Most

Is This Too Good to Be True?

- You're probably thinking, "If I ate anything in the world I wanted, I'd live on junk food and gain a ton! This is where I part ways with the authors—they're nuts!"

- It's true. At first you may eat a lot of junk food, or other forbidden (fattening) foods. But if you ALLOW yourself to do that, what you WANT will gradually change from forbidden foods to healthier and healthier foods. (Secret #6 will address nutrition.)

- Research shows that small children allowed to choose any food from a wide variety of foods (including junk food) select, on their own, a totally balanced diet over a period of time! At first, though, they, too, ate foods they previously had not been allowed to have.[25]

- Also, you will not gain an ounce from eating what you want IF you eat *only between hunger and satisfaction.*

- The amount of food you want in order to go from hunger to satisfaction is exactly the number of calories your body needs to consume to arrive at and maintain your ideal weight.

It's not *what* you eat that makes you fat— it is *how* much and *when* you eat.

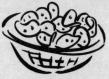

Myth → You Can't Get Fat if You Don't Eat Fat

- What do farmers fatten cows and pigs on in the Midwest? Corn and grain! There is no fat in corn or grain!

- Many people become vegetarians thinking that they will lose weight because they aren't eating animal fat or dairy products. Often they gain weight because they *eat more!* In fact, Sumo wrestlers eat mainly rice and vegetables and almost no fat. They simply eat a massive amount and sleep most of the day.[26]

- It's not *what* you eat that makes you fat. It is *when* and *how much*.

- Many wild animals who are foragers and eat mainly a vegetarian diet have an extremely high body-fat content (e.g., bears, elephants, whales, etc.).

- Other wild animals who are mainly carnivores with a high-fat diet have an extremely lean body-fat content (e.g., leopards, tigers, etc.).

- If you eat when you are not hungry, the food goes to storage (fat). And if you eat more than satisfaction, the food goes to storage (fat).

- You can gain weight on ANY food. If you eat raw vegetables beyond satisfaction, you are putting *more* food in than your body can burn, and you will gain weight. You can lose weight on *any* food. If you eat pastries, and stop at satisfaction, you are not over-loading your body, and you will lose (*if* you are overweight).

You can gain weight on *any* food.

You can lose weight on *any* food.

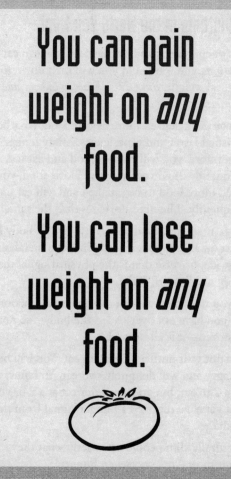

Eat Anything in the World You Want

- Between hunger and satisfaction, you can eat *anything* you want, and you will melt down to your natural weight. *But ONLY between hunger and satisfaction.*

- If you eat a denser, more caloric food, your body is satisfied faster and experiences satiety longer. Therefore, you will eat less food and eat less frequently. If you eat a lower caloric food, you will need more food to be satisfied and will eat more frequently. The net caloric result is the same!

- Also, if you put food in *only* when your body says start (at a *2*), it goes directly into the metabolic furnace, because that is the physical signal that the body needs more fuel.

- If you *stop* when your body signals satisfaction (at a *5*), you have not overloaded the body—so nothing is stored—it is all burned.

- Do not wait until a *1* or a *0* to eat. You will be *too* hungry and will definitely overeat. You must *wait* to a *2* to eat, but you also *must* eat at a *2* or you will not yet have received a hunger signal from the body.

- Naturally slim people eat exactly what they want most—but *only* when hungry!

Calories and fat grams don't count *at all* between hunger and satisfaction (a *2* and a *5*).

Successful Weight Loss Always Involves a *Limit*

- Think of all the diets you've been on (or heard of).

- People have lost weight on all of them.

- Some diets allow you to eat all the fat and protein you want but limit carbohydrates.

- Some diets allow you to eat any food, as long as you limit the calories.

- Some diets allow you to eat any food, as long as you control the combination of foods that are eaten together.

- Some diets don't care *how much* you eat as long as you limit fat grams.

- Some diets don't care *what* you eat, but they limit *when* you can eat. For example, only fruit in the morning, nothing between meals, and nothing after dinner.

Your new limits are to eat whatever you want, but *only* between hunger and satisfaction.

Never Deprive

- **Deprivation creates overeating.**

- Deprivation leaves you feeling physiologically and psychologically unsatisfied.

- Even normal-weight people, normal eaters, overeat at Thanksgiving and Christmas. Why? *Because they get those special foods only two times a year.* Consequently, the rest of the year they are deprived of those foods.

- What is your favorite food at Thanksgiving? What if you allowed yourself to have that food at least once a week all year long. Could it possibly trigger overeating on Thanksgiving Day? Not likely!

- The only way you will stop overeating is if you promise yourself that you can have more of that tempting food, and that you can have it *every* time, if you want, until the end of your life!

- **Do not deprive yourself ever again.**

When you *can't* have something, you only want it more.

Carry a Favorite Binge Food With You Everywhere

- You usually binge on foods that you don't ever *allow* yourself to have.

- Even though you eat them while binging, you don't feel *entitled* to be eating them because you are not yet slim.

- So you can never truly enjoy these foods or eat them with *permission!* By making them "bad" or "illegal," you give them tremendous power!

- Do not think about a pink elephant. See! The minute you are told *not to*, that's exactly what pops into your mind!

- The minute you tell yourself you CAN'T have something, that is all you can think about! It now controls you rather than the other way around.

- We know it sounds paradoxical, but in order to stop binging, you must give yourself *permission* to binge on the most appealing food possible.

- Take a favorite binge food with you everywhere, even to bed! Every time *you are hungry*, have some (if that is what you want), and eat it consciously.

The best way to avoid temptation is to give in to it!

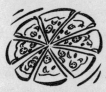

Deliberately Have a Conscious Binge

- Since you are carrying a binge food everywhere, you may be afraid you will binge on it.

- *That's OK!* You are going to learn *how* to do a binge differently! So it has no emotional or caloric consequences!

- DO A CONSCIOUS BINGE:

  - *Pick the tastiest food possible!*

  - *Sit down.*

  - *Give every bite your* total *attention.*

  - *Enjoy—fork down after every bite.*

  - *Eat as much as you* want.

  - *Notice how your body feels before, during, and after the binge.*

  - *If you overate, all* you have to do is *wait until you're hungry again* to eat again, and your body will have burned up any excess calories!

  - *Don't worry—you will not receive the hunger signal again until the excess calories are burned.*

To binge consciously is to become free of binging.

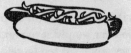

Fill Your House with All of Your Favorite Foods

- You believe that the better the food, the more you are likely to overeat it.

- In fact, the opposite is true. Mediocre food causes overeating, You keep eating more and more of it, searching for satisfaction.

- You can never get enough of what you don't really want![27]

- The only way you will overeat a great food is if:

  - *You don't have enough of that food in your daily life.* Solution? **Buy more of it.**

  - *You plan to deprive yourself of great foods as soon as you finish eating this meal.* Solution? **Never deprive yourself again.**

- If it is too scary to go to the grocery store and stock up on *everything* you've ever wanted, do it one food at a time.

- That means, if you want potato chips, buy ten large bags, and *keep* your supply at ten large bags. (There's *no way* you'll eat ten large bags at one sitting, no matter how hard you try!)

- When potato chips lose their power, add another food in quantity. But don't get rid of the potato chips! Keep adding foods—no subtracting!

One of the fastest ways to gain weight is to settle for second best.

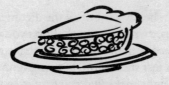

SECRET 5:
Eat What You Want Most

WEEK-FIVE ASSIGNMENTS

1. Continue to keep your Body Awareness Log.

2. Carry a favorite binge food with you everywhere this week. Every time you are *hungry*, you may have it, as long as you eat it *consciously*. At the end of the week, enter the results of this experiment in this section.

3. Deliberately have a conscious binge (described on page 164). Enter the results of this experiment in this section.

4. At the end of this week, fill your house with all of your favorite foods. If that is too scary, add one "forbidden" food a week, in a large quantity, until gradually you have desensitized yourself to all foods.

5. Write down below a list of all the dieting, restricting, or weight-control efforts you've experimented with in your life. Describe the results, not just short term, but long term. Did you gain the weight back? Did you gain even more weight back than you originally lost? The purpose of this exercise is to remind you how restricting and controlling hasn't worked for you, and to encourage you to risk taking the steps assigned this week.

SECRET 5:
Eat What You Want Most

example
Body Awareness Log

Check off what you did. In hunger columns, enter the number that applies.

Time	Sat Down	No Distractions	Fork Down	No Judgment	Hunger Level Start	Comfort Level Stop	Fist Size	Ate What Wanted Most?
6:00AM	no	no	✔	judged	2	4	✔	yes
8:30AM	✔	✔	✔	judged	3	5	✔	yes
12:00PM	✔	✔	no	✔	2	5	✔	no
6:30PM	✔	✔	✔	✔	2	5	✔	no
9:00PM	no	no	no	judged	5	7	no	yes

What Did You Learn from This?	I feel guilty when I eat exactly what I want because I can't believe fattening food won't make me fat!

SECRET 5:
Eat What You Want Most

Body Awareness Log
DAY ONE

Check off what you did. In hunger columns, enter the number that applies.

Time	Sat Down	No Distractions	Fork Down	No Judgment	Hunger Level Start	Comfort Level Stop	Fist Size	Ate What Wanted Most?

What Did You Learn from This?

SECRET 5:
Eat What You Want Most

Body Awareness Log
DAY TWO

Check off what you did. In hunger columns, enter the number that applies.

Time	Sat Down	No Distractions	Fork Down	No Judgment	Hunger Level Start	Comfort Level Stop	Fist Size	Ate What Wanted Most?

What Did You Learn from This?

SECRET 5:
Eat What You Want Most

Body Awareness Log
DAY THREE

Check off what you did. In hunger columns, enter the number that applies.

Time	Sat Down	No Distractions	Fork Down	No Judgment	Hunger Level Start	Comfort Level Stop	Fist Size	Ate What Wanted Most?

What Did You Learn from This?

SECRET 5:
Eat What You Want Most

Body Awareness Log
DAY FOUR

Check off what you did. In hunger columns, enter the number that applies.

Time	Sat Down	No Distractions	Fork Down	No Judgment	Hunger Level Start	Comfort Level Stop	Fist Size	Ate What Wanted Most?

What Did You Learn from This?

SECRET 5:
Eat What You Want Most

Body Awareness Log
DAY FIVE

Check off what you did. In hunger columns, enter the number that applies.

Time	Sat Down	No Distractions	Fork Down	No Judgment	Hunger Level Start	Comfort Level Stop	Fist Size	Ate What Wanted Most?

What Did You Learn from This?

SECRET 5:
Eat What You Want Most

Body Awareness Log
DAY SIX

Check off what you did. In hunger columns, enter the number that applies.

Time	Sat Down	No Distractions	Fork Down	No Judgment	Hunger Level Start	Comfort Level Stop	Fist Size	Ate What Wanted Most?

What Did You Learn from This?

SECRET 5:
Eat What You Want Most

Body Awareness Log
DAY SEVEN

Check off what you did. In hunger columns, enter the number that applies.

Time	Sat Down	No Distractions	Fork Down	No Judgment	Hunger Level Start	Comfort Level Stop	Fist Size	Ate What Wanted Most?

What Did You Learn from This?

Carrying-Your-Favorite-Binge-Food-With-You-Everywhere Experiment

(DESCRIBED ON PAGE 162)

1. What were your fears when you started this experiment?

2. Did your fears come true?

3. What did you learn from this experiment?

4. Were there any surprises?

Have-A-Conscious-Binge Experiment

(DESCRIBED ON PAGE 164)

1. How did it feel to you to binge deliberately and consciously?

2. What did you learn from this experiment?

3. The best way to break a binge in the future is simply to begin doing the binge CONSCIOUSLY at the moment you become aware of wanting to stop binging. You cannot be unconscious (binging) and conscious (aware) at the same time.

Fill-Your-House-With-All-of-Your-Favorite-Foods Experiment

(DESCRIBED ON PAGE 166)

1. How did it feel to stock up on whatever you wanted at the grocery store?

2. What was scary, and what was reassuring about it?

3. What are your fears about having all this food in your house?

4. How can you reassure yourself?

CHAPTER 9

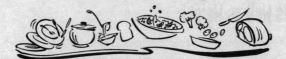

SECRET 6:

Notice How Your

Body Feels *After*

Eating

Your Body Regulates Nutrition as Well as Weight

- After you practice conscious eating for a while, what *you* most *want* to eat, and what your *body* most *wants* to eat, will become one and the same.

- But, if you've ever dieted or deprived yourself of food, you will first need to physically and emotionally recover from the effects of this deprivation before you will be *able* to listen to and honor what your *body* wants to eat.

- The way you recover is to allow yourself to eat *anything*—but only between hunger and satisfaction. You cannot make up for 20 years of deprivation by eating enough food *today* to compensate for all that you didn't give yourself in the past.

- But you *can* give yourself *any* food at the appropriate time of hunger, and soon deprivation will no longer be an issue.

- Your body tells you what it wants to eat through appetite cravings and through how your body feels after eating or drinking.

What you most
want to eat and
what your body
most wants to eat
will gradually become
one and the same.

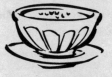

Give Your Body What It *Most* Wants to Eat

- Perfect eating for ideal health and weight depends on your continuing to fine-tune your awareness of how your body likes the foods you are putting into it.

- The ways to make a good food-to-body match are:

  - *What are you craving when you are hungry?*

  - *If you eat it, does it taste great? If it's a body craving, the food will taste phenomenal.*

  - *How does your body feel 30 minutes to a few hours after eating the food?*

  - *If the food was a good body match, you will feel great.*

  - *If the food was a bad match, you'll have acid, gas, pain, nausea, discomfort, etc.*

- There are only two reasons your body will feel bad after eating when you are hungry:

  - *You made a bad match, or a bad combination of foods.*

  - *You ate too much food, even if it was a good match.*

You cannot *tell* your body what to do and *listen* to it at the same time.

Identify Body Cravings

- If you are sure you are hungry, but not sure what you most want, shut your eyes and imagine asking your stomach to signal its preference among these choices. Do you want something that is:

  – *Hot or Cold?*

  – *Hearty or Light?*

  – *Creamy or Crunchy?*

  – *Sweet, Sour, or Salty?*

  – *Spicy or Bland?*

  – *Protein, Carbohydrate, or Fat?*

- For example, as you imagine these different sensations in your stomach, your responses may be that you want something hot, hearty, creamy, bland, salty, and carbohydrate filled. Ask yourself what would be a good match. Perhaps oatmeal occurs to you. Eat it and notice how it agrees with your body afterwards.

- Your body normally will not crave multiple foods at once. When you are nutritionally in need of something, that is what you will crave and what will feel good in your body AFTER eating it.

Usually a *body* craving tells you what you want *before* you see or smell food.

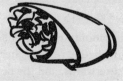

"Won't I Crave the Food I'm Addicted To?"

- If you are addicted to a certain food, you will certainly crave it. But, if it is not what your body wants to eat, your body will not feel good after eating it.

- Vikki was addicted to sugar for 23 years. Even while calorie counting, she would eat as much sugar as she could. She loved the way it tasted and how it made her feel while she was eating it.

- But, once she started to notice how she felt *afterwards*, she realized she always got a sugar rush at first, and then a drop in energy and a feeling of nausea. She would then drink three to four cups of coffee to try to counteract the energy loss.

- By staying conscious while eating the sugar, when that was what she wanted to eat, and by noticing how her body felt *afterwards*, she became less and less attracted to sugar.

- She knows she can *have* sugar. It's not an illegal food. In fact, she keeps many sweets in her house.

- Every time her mouth wants just sugar for a meal, her body immediately reminds her of how terrible she will feel afterwards, and the desire fades away.

- She's also learned that she can have small amounts of sweets following real food, with no ill effects.

Feeding an addictive
craving leaves your body
feeling bad afterwards.

Feeding a body
craving leaves your body
feeling good afterwards.

Food Combinations

- If you eat a meal and *know* you did not overeat, but feel bad afterwards, you may want to experiment with eating the various foods at the meal separately or in different combinations to find out what works for your body.

- For example, perhaps you had half a burger, half a piece of pie, and a cup of coffee, then had a stomachache afterwards. Experiment with different combinations to find the culprit. For example:

  > *burger and pie.........body felt good*
  > – *burger and coffee.....body felt bad*
  > – *pie and coffee...........body felt bad*

  Hence, the culprit here is the coffee.

- One client discovered that her body didn't like coffee, but she loved the smell and taste of coffee. By experimenting, she discovered certain brands of coffee that agreed with her. She also discovered that if she drank a large glass of water with her cup of coffee, she felt fine afterwards.

- By paying attention and by experimenting, you will discover exactly which foods, which combination of foods, which brands of foods and drinks, even which fast foods agree with you and which ones don't.

- You will become an expert on your own body and how to feed yourself to feel and look wonderful.

- Since you are allowed to eat anything and never deprive yourself, you will soon find yourself making choices that make you feel better and better in your body. The lighter and more energetic you look and feel, the more you know that you are making good nutritional matches.

You can eat *any* food; you just have to discover *how* to eat it so it agrees with your body.

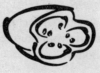

Every Body Is Different

- Your body will tell you how to eat perfectly *for you* and no one else.

- What makes you feel best may not exactly match general nutritional guidelines.

- For example, you may feel best on many small carbohydrate meals a day. Someone else may feel best on two larger high-protein meals a day, and yet another person may feel best on a higher-fat diet.

- Whatever makes your body feel great is what's best for you and will create your uniquely, ideal-looking, healthy body.

- Try it, test it, trust it, and see how you feel!

How your body wishes to eat will differ from other people's bodies.

The Role of Liquids

- Just as you have learned to eat for hunger, now you need to learn to drink for thirst.

- You may drink when you are hungry, to try to delay your hunger. Don't. When you are hungry, eat! If you are feeling *actual* hunger, liquid will only temporarily delay the return of the hunger feeling.

- You may think you are hungry when you are actually thirsty. For example, one client thought he woke up starving every morning, but discovered he was thirsty rather than hungry. He discovered this by having juice, water, or coffee, and realized that he didn't feel actual hunger until 10 or 11 A.M.

- If you drink liquid with your meals, it may make it difficult to identify hunger and satisfaction signals.

- Don't think that low-calorie or no-calorie liquids have no impact on how your body feels. *Everything has an impact!* If you stopped eating at satisfaction, and put a cup of black coffee on top of your meal, you don't add any extra calories, but you just moved your body into discomfort, which is always inappropriate.

- If you like liquid during or at the end of your meal, *leave room!* Just recognize that it will occupy part of the space you could have devoted to food.

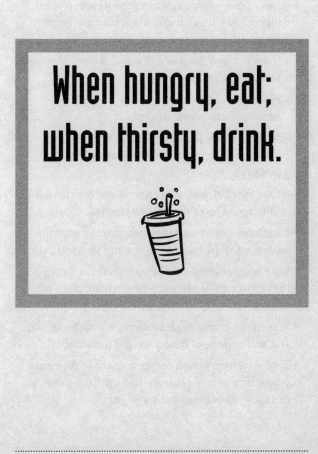

When hungry, eat; when thirsty, drink.

The Pleasure/Pain Principle

- Pain and pleasure are both feedback signals that are essential to your survival.

- People born without pain receptors are in great danger. They don't know when they are getting hurt.

  - *If you put your hand in a fire, it will hurt.* Message? **Don't do that anymore.**

  - *Pleasure is also a message.* Message? **Do more of that.**

  - *Food tastes fabulous when you are really hungry.* Message? **Do more of that (eat only when hungry).**

  - *Your body feels pain if you get too empty or too full?* Message? **Don't do that anymore!**

- Your body communicates with you through the sensations of physical pleasure and physical pain.

- Your body communicates with you also through the sensations of physical comfort and physical discomfort.

- Stay in the comfort/pleasure zone with food, and you will no longer have a weight problem!

- Your weight problem comes from only depriving yourself of *enough* pleasure and joy from your eating! Follow pleasure; avoid pain.

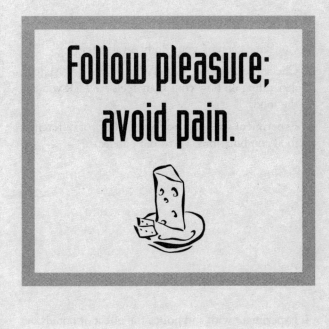

Follow pleasure;
avoid pain.

SECRET 6:
Notice How Your Body Feels *After* Eating

WEEK-SIX ASSIGNMENTS

1. Continue keeping your Body Awareness Log.

2. Check the columns "Good Match" or "Bad Match" depending on how your body feels AFTER you eat the food.

3. Experiment with and notice the effect of different food combinations. What did you learn?

4. Experiment with and notice the effect of liquids on your body. What did you learn?

SECRET 6:
Notice How Your Body Feels *After* Eating

example

Body Awareness Log

Check off what you did. In hunger columns, enter the number that applies.

Time	Sat Down	No Distractions	Fist Size	Fork Down	No Judgment	Hunger Level Start	Comfort Level Stop	Good Match	Bad Match
7:00AM	✓	✓	✓	✓	✓	2	5	no	✓
10:00AM	✓	✓	✓	✓	✓	2	5	✓	no
7:00PM	✓	no	no	no	no	1	7	no	✓

What Did You Learn from This?	I learned that my <u>body</u> doesn't like coffee. If I get too hungry, I eat too much. My body hates feeling too full.

SECRET 6:
Notice How Your Body Feels *After* Eating

Body Awareness Log
DAY ONE

Check off what you did. In hunger columns, enter the number that applies.

Time	Sat Down	No Distractions	Fist Size	Fork Down	No Judgment	Hunger Level Start	Comfort Level Stop	Good Match	Bad Match

What Did You Learn from This?

SECRET 6:
Notice How Your Body Feels *After* Eating

Body Awareness Log
DAY TWO

Check off what you did. In hunger columns, enter the number that applies.

Time	Sat Down	No Distractions	Fist Size	Fork Down	No Judgment	Hunger Level Start	Comfort Level Stop	Good Match	Bad Match

What Did You Learn from This?

SECRET 6:
Notice How Your Body Feels *After* Eating

Body Awareness Log
DAY THREE

Check off what you did. In hunger columns, enter the number that applies.

Time	Sat Down	No Distractions	Fist Size	Fork Down	No Judgment	Hunger Level Start	Comfort Level Stop	Good Match	Bad Match

What Did You Learn from This?

SECRET 6:
Notice How Your Body Feels *After* Eating

Body Awareness Log
DAY FOUR

Check off what you did. In hunger columns, enter the number that applies.

Time	Sat Down	No Distractions	Fist Size	Fork Down	No Judgment	Hunger Level Start	Comfort Level Stop	Good Match	Bad Match

What Did You Learn from This?

SECRET 6:
Notice How Your Body Feels *After* Eating

Body Awareness Log
DAY FIVE

Check off what you did. In hunger columns, enter the number that applies.

Time	Sat Down	No Distractions	Fist Size	Fork Down	No Judgment	Hunger Level Start	Comfort Level Stop	Good Match	Bad Match

What Did You Learn from This?

SECRET 6:
Notice How Your Body Feels *After* Eating

Body Awareness Log
DAY SIX

Check off what you did. In hunger columns, enter the number that applies.

Time	Sat Down	No Distractions	Fist Size	Fork Down	No Judgment	Hunger Level Start	Comfort Level Stop	Good Match	Bad Match

What Did You Learn from This?

SECRET 6:
Notice How Your Body Feels *After* Eating

Body Awareness Log
DAY SEVEN

Check off what you did. In hunger columns, enter the number that applies.

Time	Sat Down	No Distractions	Fist Size	Fork Down	No Judgment	Hunger Level Start	Comfort Level Stop	Good Match	Bad Match

What Did You Learn from This?

Additional Notes for the Week

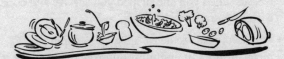

CHAPTER 10

SECRET 7:
Honor Your Feelings; Don't Bury Them Under Food

Eating Has Been Your Life Preserver

- If you have ever eaten for emotional reasons, eating has sustained you and helped you survive and cope with life's stresses and crises.

- You don't just decide to "give up" a coping mechanism. You first must outgrow the need for it.

- Food may have been there for you when nothing else was. It may have been a source of comfort and stability.

- Food has never been your enemy! Eating has always been an attempt to nurture yourself in some way.

- It is just a bad match. If you're bored, you need stimulation, not cheesecake. If you're sad, you need to grieve, not to eat pizza.

- You aren't a bad person with low willpower simply because you've eaten to cope! You would have taken a better alternative if you had one.

- The problem is: long ago all of your hungers became confused into one signal—the signal for food!

- By now you know what physical hunger feels like. That is the first step to untangling your hungers.

- Be grateful for all the ways eating has helped you survive.

We will not take away your life preserver.

We will teach you how to swim!

The Overeating Spiral

- As an emotional eater, you *learned* that if you had an *uncomfortable feeling*, eating would make it go away.

- When you were little, the eating loop stopped right there.

- As you got older, you learned to *judge* yourself as a bad person for eating—especially if you ate for emotional reasons.

- Judging yourself led to a new uncomfortable feeling, which led to more eating, more judgment, more eating, and so on.

- So, eating *once* over an uncomfortable feeling triggers a downward spiral of shame, self-disgust, and more overeating.

- The first place to practice breaking this loop is to *refuse to judge yourself*, no matter what you do with food.

- If you do not judge yourself, you will prevent a great deal of overeating.

- No matter what, how much, or for what reason you eat, *accept* that it was necessary, make it OK with yourself, and notice what happened. Then move on.

- Say to yourself, "That's OK, honey, you truly must have needed to do that!"

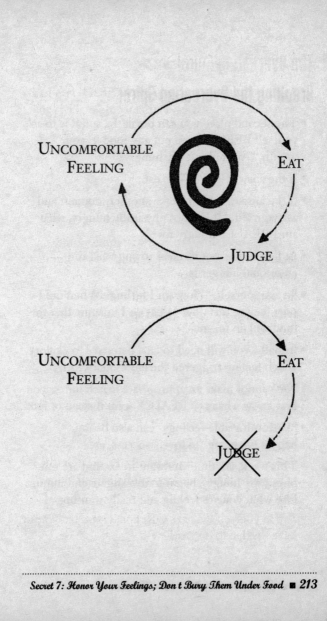

UNCOMFORTABLE
FEELING

EAT

JUDGE

UNCOMFORTABLE
FEELING

EAT

JUDGE

Breaking the Overeating Spiral

- The second place you can break the spiral is to ask yourself BEFORE you put any food in your mouth, "Am I physically hungry?"

- If the answer is "Yes," go eat!

- If the answer is "No," take another moment and ask yourself, "If I'm not physically hungry, what am I REALLY hungry for?"

- At first it may not be clear to you what the emotional hunger is.

- So ask yourself, "How am I feeling? When did I start feeling this way? What do I imagine that this food will do for me?"

- Initially, you will need to be a detective to explore which feeling triggered the emotional eating.

- You cannot make an appropriate match unless you first know what you REALLY want instead of food.

- "Uncomfortable feelings" can also be joy, happiness, being "in love," success, etc.

- This week, anytime you want to eat and are not physically hungry, begin to investigate and inquire into what you are feeling and really wanting.

Go Back to Your Feelings

BREAK

UNCOMFORTABLE
FEELING

EAT

Non-Hunger Eating

- Eating for *any* reason other than physical hunger is non-hunger eating.

- Non-hunger eating is what *creates* weight gain.

- Non-hunger eating is *always* your desire or need for something else besides food.

- You eat when you are not hungry in order to become unconscious, in order not to feel those uncomfortable feelings or needs anymore.

- In this way you use food as a drug—to go numb.

- *And it works!* Food numbs you and comforts you *just enough* to *continue* doing what is causing the uncomfortable feeling in the first place.

- Why would you want to continue doing what is uncomfortable? Perhaps because your deeper hungers or problems feel too big, too unresolvable, or too painful to face? Perhaps you don't feel you deserve to have a better job, mate, or friends—or, that change is too scary.

- Then, you eat not to make yourself happy, but to tolerate being so unhappy. And this seems to work—you are able to cope.

- What are the reasons you can think of that cause you to engage in non-hunger eating? In each case, what feeling or unmet need is the food allowing you to tolerate?

Non-hunger eating allows you to tolerate the intolerable.

How Food Keeps You Stuck

- Overeating *prevents* you from getting what you really want out of life.

- It numbs you *just enough* to cause you to settle for less than you deserve.

- As long as food is your lover, you'll never find your ideal relationship.

- As long as food is your companion, you'll never discover true friends.

- As long as food is your reward, you'll never learn what truly pleasures you.

- As long as food is used to fill the hole in your heart, you'll never fulfill your potential.

- The hole in your heart is not there by accident. It is there to send helpful messages to you about what you *need* to be truly happy. These messages cannot be ignored forever or buried by overeating.

- The goal is not to fill the hole in order to get on with your life.

- FILLING THE HOLE IN YOUR HEART IS WHAT YOUR LIFE IS ABOUT!

- How has eating become a substitute for living your dreams? It's OK to grieve. The next step shows you the way out of being stuck.

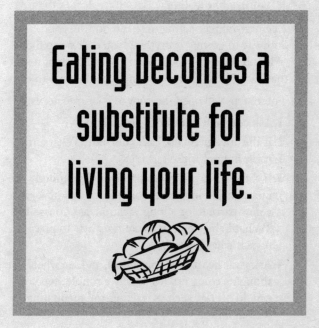

Eating becomes a substitute for living your life.

The Non-Hunger Eating Urge Is Your Best Friend!

- You are so lucky to have an eating problem! The moment you want to do non-hunger eating, you now know that what you really want is to feed a deeper need or feeling.

- The non-hunger eating urge can now be your doorway to getting everything you ever wanted out of life. It physically points out your important needs that have been masked until now by the urge to eat.

- These steps will open the door to your true needs:

  1. Ask yourself: "Am I physically hungry?"

  2. If the answer is "no," ask yourself, "What am I *really* hungry for?"

  3. If the answer is something big and seemingly unattainable in that moment, such as a new job, a new partner, or a long vacation, ask yourself, "What baby step can I take *right now* to give myself what I want?"

  4. Ask your heart (not your head), and see what thoughts come up. It's usually a simple step you can do NOW, such as walking and meditating for ten minutes.

  5. *Do it!* With one baby step at a time, larger needs and wishes will get filled, sooner than you could possibly imagine. You *must* feed your important needs and wishes *now*.

  6. If it takes more than 15 minutes or $15, it is not a baby step.[28]

Anytime you want to eat when you are not hungry, it is just an "ignored" part of you asking for nourishment.

The Core Problem Is: Lack of Self-Love

- Do you trust your body, your feelings, yourself?

- Probably not, because if you did, it would be impossible to have an eating problem!

- How did this lack of self-trust occur?

- You were born trusting yourself, but with a natural hunger for love. You were completely dependent on your parents to meet your needs. You looked up to them for love and approval. Did you get enough love to feel totally lovable?

- Probably not. Hardly anyone does! So you looked next to another source; friends and teachers. Were you ever popular enough to feel completely lovable?

- Probably not. Hardly anyone does! So you turned next to our great cultural romance myth. You were missing your soulmate, your other half! Did you ever find a soulmate able to *complete* you?

- In each of these cases, you were looking for love in all the wrong places—*OUTSIDE OF YOURSELF!* You don't have a food addiction, you have an approval addiction.

- When you couldn't get enough love or approval, you picked a substitute—food, drugs, work, sex, power.

- Whose approval have you sought and do you seek now? Do you try to change yourself to please them?

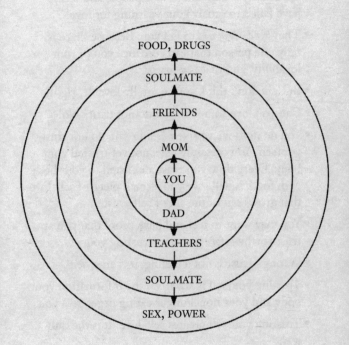

FOOD, DRUGS

SOULMATE

FRIENDS

MOM

YOU

DAD

TEACHERS

SOULMATE

SEX, POWER

You Cannot Love Someone You Do Not Trust

- It's *wonderful* that all of those people and things have failed to satisfy your yearning for love!

- They were *designed* to fail you. Because there is only one person that can convince you of your lovability, and that is *yourself!*

- But *you* don't think you're totally lovable, right?

- Can you love someone you do not trust? No!

- You do not love yourself *because* you do not trust yourself. You certainly have not yet trusted your body. Every time you trust and listen to your body with food, it will give you a small piece of self-love that grows out of the act of self-trust.

- You may want to feel and have proof that you are trustworthy *before* you start trusting yourself.

- Wrong. Trust is not a feeling; it is an *action!*

- Trusting yourself is *acting* on the information your body and your non-hunger eating urges give you.

- Trusting yourself creates self-love. It is the only way.

- Practice trusting your body, your feelings, and yourself in all parts of your life.

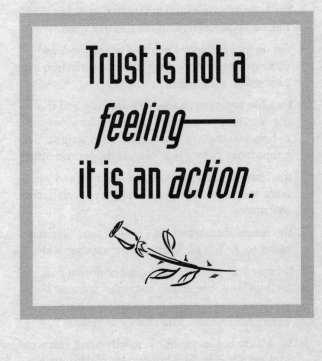

Trust is not a *feeling*— it is an *action*.

The Stages of Becoming a Normal Eater

1. You distinguish between physical and emotional hunger and start making appropriate matches.

2. You begin to get in touch with your feelings and begin to honor them.

3. You learn to stop eating at satisfaction rather than full, and you feel light at the end of a meal.

4. You no longer deprive yourself of any food, and you experience more pleasure and satisfaction with eating than ever before.

5. Your life begins to change dramatically, and this may feel very chaotic and upsetting. You may eat to help you cope. You may gain some weight, temporarily, before you lose weight permanently.

6. You learn to judge yourself less and less, and you learn how to encourage and support yourself more and more.

7. You notice that you spend a lot less time thinking about food. You are learning to trust your body.

8. Because you are listening to and honoring your feelings, and listening to and honoring your body, you are eating less and less frequently for emotional reasons. This change is gradual.

9. Your body begins to shrink, mostly when you aren't looking. One day you notice your clothes are all loose. And as you move to a smaller size, one day you notice that they are all loose again. THIS HAPPENS FASTEST WHEN YOUR FOCUS IS ON LISTENING TO AND TRUSTING

YOUR BODY AND YOURSELF, RATHER THAN WHEN YOUR FOCUS IS ON WEIGHT LOSS. FOCUSING ON WEIGHT LOSS SLOWS YOU DOWN.

10. One day you realize that your body has stabilized. You can eat exactly what you want when you are hungry, and your weight only fluctuates slightly. You look great, you feel great, and you hardly ever think about food except when your body is hungry.

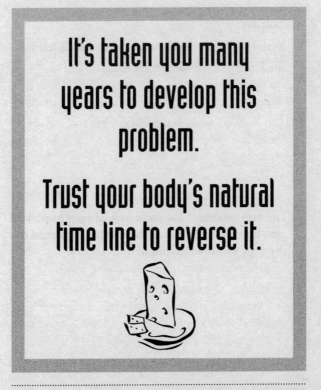

It's taken you many years to develop this problem.

Trust your body's natural time line to reverse it.

SECRET 7:
Honor Your Feelings;
Don't Bury Them Under Food

WEEK-SEVEN ASSIGNMENTS

1. Continue to eat consciously in all the ways you have learned so far.

2. Keep the Body/Feeling Awareness Log each day.

3. At the end of the week, write down which feelings triggered non-hunger eating.

4. Did you take any baby steps to feed your important non-hunger needs and wishes? What happened to the urge to eat when you did?

SECRET 7:
Honor Your Feelings;
Don't Bury Them Under Food

example

Body Awareness Log

Check off what you did each time, and record any appropriate comments.

Time	Hunger Level at Start	Comfort Level at Stop	No Judgment	What Feeling	If You Ate for Non-Hunger Reasons, What Did You *Really* Want? Did You Take a Baby Step Toward Satisfying Your *Real* Hunger?
7:00AM	2	5	✓	fine	
10:00AM	4	6	judged	rushed	Wanted a break—ate a doughnut instead. Step: Walked around the building for fresh air.
1:00PM	2	5	✓	neutral	
4:00PM	4	7	✓	tired	Wanted energy: Took a nap.
9:00PM	2	7	judged	lonely	Wanted companionship: Called a friend.

SECRET 7:
Honor Your Feelings;
Don't Bury Them Under Food

Body Awareness Log
DAY ONE

Check off what you did each time, and record any appropriate comments.

Time	Hunger Level at Start	Comfort Level at Stop	No Judgment	What Feeling	If You Ate for Non-Hunger Reasons, What Did You *Really* Want? Did You Take a Baby Step Toward Satisfying Your *Real* Hunger?

SECRET 7:
Honor Your Feelings;
Don't Bury Them Under Food

Body Awareness Log
DAY TWO

Check off what you did each time, and record any appropriate comments.

Time	Hunger Level at Start	Comfort Level at Stop	No Judgment	What Feeling	If You Ate for Non-Hunger Reasons, What Did You *Really* Want? Did You Take a Baby Step Toward Satisfying Your *Real* Hunger?

SECRET 7:
Honor Your Feelings;
Don't Bury Them Under Food

Body Awareness Log
DAY THREE

Check off what you did each time, and record any appropriate comments.

Time	Hunger Level at Start	Comfort Level at Stop	No Judgment	What Feeling	If You Ate for Non-Hunger Reasons, What Did You *Really* Want? Did You Take a Baby Step Toward Satisfying Your *Real* Hunger?

SECRET 7:
Honor Your Feelings;
Don't Bury Them Under Food

Body Awareness Log
DAY FOUR

Check off what you did each time, and record any appropriate comments.

Time	Hunger Level at Start	Comfort Level at Stop	No Judgment	What Feeling	If You Ate For Non-Hunger Reasons, What Did You *Really* Want? Did You Take a Baby Step Toward Satisfying Your *Real* Hunger?

SECRET 7:
Honor Your Feelings;
Don't Bury Them Under Food

Body Awareness Log
DAY FIVE

Check off what you did each time, and record any appropriate comments.

Time	Hunger Level at Start	Comfort Level at Stop	No Judgment	What Feeling	If You Ate for Non-Hunger Reasons, What Did You *Really* Want? Did You Take a Baby Step Toward Satisfying Your *Real* Hunger?

SECRET 7:
Honor Your Feelings;
Don't Bury Them Under Food

Body Awareness Log
DAY SIX

Check off what you did each time, and record any appropriate comments.

Time	Hunger Level at Start	Comfort Level at Stop	No Judgment	What Feeling	If You Ate for Non-Hunger Reasons, What Did You *Really* Want? Did You Take a Baby Step Toward Satisfying Your *Real* Hunger?

SECRET 7:
Honor Your Feelings;
Don't Bury Them Under Food

Body Awareness Log
DAY SEVEN

Check off what you did each time, and record any appropriate comments.

Time	Hunger Level at Start	Comfort Level at Stop	No Judgment	What Feeling	If You Ate For Non-Hunger Reasons, What Did You *Really* Want? Did You Take a Baby Step Toward Satisfying Your *Real* Hunger?

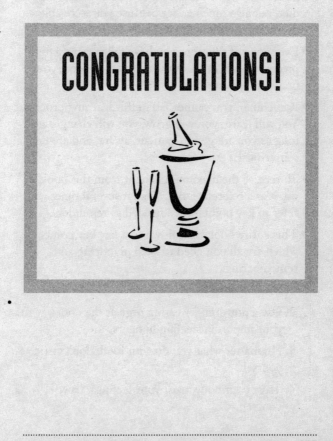

CONGRATULATIONS!

Congratulations!

- You have spent the last seven weeks learning how to listen to your body and your feelings. Be proud of yourself.

- In many ways, this has been much harder than a diet, but also much easier because you were able to eat exactly what you wanted!

- Every one of the steps you have taken represents a profound shift in the way you relate to food, your body, and yourself.

- Remember, you cannot fail in this learning process. You will learn, you will grow, you will change, as long as you are gentle, patient, aware, and are not self-critical.

- To receive the maximum benefit from this book, use it as a reference tool. Read it several times and refer to key points when needed as reminders.

- This entire book boils down to a few key points, which are all you need to keep practicing and remembering.

  1. Eat consciously.

  2. Use a non-hunger eating urge as the doorway to your important feeling hungers.

  3. No matter what you do with food, don't criticize yourself.

  4. Trust your body, trust your feelings, trust yourself.

Key Points

1. Eat consciously
2. Don't judge
3. Trust yourself
4. Trust your feelings

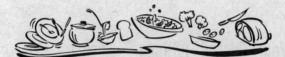

CHAPTER 11

To Be Slim for Life, You Must Adopt the Attitudes of the Naturally Slim

Your "Control" Attitude—Lose It

- The next big step on your path to freedom from eating issues is to adopt some new attitudes.

- It is your *ATTITUDE* of self-criticism and control that creates problems with food.

- "Controlling" your body and your food through diets, excessive exercise, or controlled weight management does not work.

- Attempting to control your body and food (i.e., diets or restricting food) only leads to the reaction of being "out of control" (overeating).

- Your goal is to get off the control/out-of-control pendulum (yo-yo dieting). Your goal is to operate with an entirely new state of mind—that is, one of *trust*.

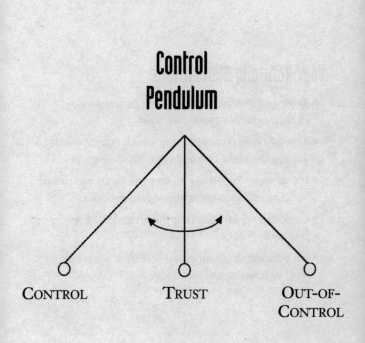

Control
Pendulum

CONTROL   TRUST   OUT-OF-
                                              CONTROL

Your Naturally Slim Attitude

- Trust and control have nothing in common. In fact, *control cancels out trust.*

- The key is to trust only that which is trustworthy. Trust your body and not your mind.

- If you want something to control, focus your need to "control" into controlling your attitude.

- Concentrate on adopting the attitude of the Naturally Slim.

- An attitude shift will create a shift in your eating and, ultimately, in your body.

Your naturally slim attitude will create a naturally slim body.

Be Kind and Compassionate with Yourself

- It's not what you *DO* with food that counts.

- It's how you *VIEW* what you do with food that counts.

- No matter what you just did with food, *VIEW* your actions with:

  - *Acceptance.*

  - *Compassion.*

  - *Awareness.*

  - *Permission.*

  - *Letting Go.*[29]

- If you adopt these attitudes, everything about your eating will change.

- No matter what "mistake" you think you have made, say only "That's OK, Honey" to yourself, and go on.

Say only: "That's OK, Honey!"

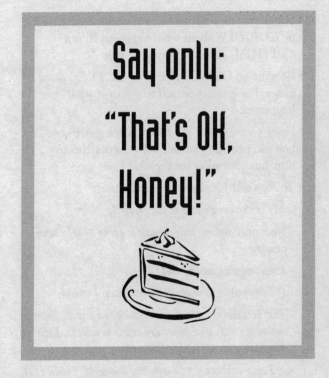

Be Curious, Not Critical

- Whenever non-hunger eating occurs (and it *will!*), be CURIOUS about what triggered it, not CRITICAL about "blowing it again."

- Become an OBJECTIVE DETECTIVE, not a judge. Look into yourself to discover what happened.

- Once you uncover the real non-hunger trigger, you can provide yourself with alternatives to non-hunger eating for the next time.

- To stop self-judgment, say to yourself:

  - *My* body *knows how to eat perfectly.*

  - Recognizing *my body signals is going to take some practice.*

  - I am *learning as fast as I can.*

  - *If I were* able *to make changes faster, I would.*

  - *Just because my* mind *can understand a step, doesn't mean my body and heart are ready to take it. I will be kind and compassionate and patient with myself.*

  - *If I ever overeat, I will only say to myself, "That's OK, honey. I wonder why that happened?"*

Ask Only:

"I wonder why that happened?"

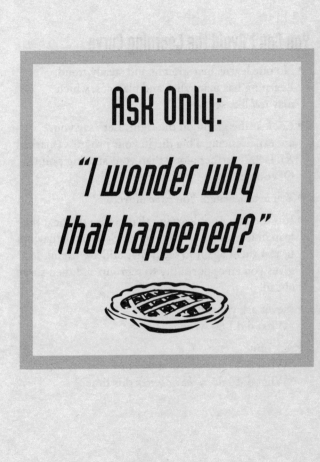

You Can't Avoid the Learning Curve

- No one learns in a straight and steady trend. Learning has many dips and plateaus, which may *feel* like setbacks.

- Look at the graph on the right. Let's say you are experiencing a big dip in your progress (marked X). Is "X" further along than your starting point? Of course!

- You *have* learned. You *have* moved.

- It is the nature of learning that before the next big leap in learning, you often go back to old behaviors to test them again to see if they still are useful. It gives you an opportunity to regroup and then surge ahead.

- Never ask yourself:
  "What did I do wrong?"

- Ask only:
  "What did I *learn* from this?" or
  "What did I do *right* or *better* this time?"

Learning Curve

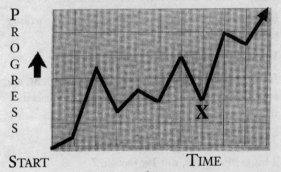

Have Endless Patience

- How much patience do you have with a baby learning to talk?

- You have to become a baby again and learn body trust, which is completely alien to you right now.

- How much TIME and SUPPORT are you willing to offer yourself?

- You ARE learning as fast as you can.

- An atmosphere of nurturance, encouragement, and acceptance will cause you to blossom the fastest.

- Your thoughts are your atmosphere.

- Think: "Evolution, not Revolution."

- Think: "Progress, not Perfection."

- Think: "Every Journey Begins with a Single Step."

- Remember: "The Race Goes Not to the Swift, But to Those Who Keep on Running."

Returning to your
naturally slim self
requires a cup of
knowledge, a barrel of
compassion, and an
ocean of patience.[30]

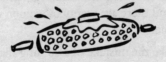

Accept and Celebrate Your Body

- By comparing yourself to the cultural standards of beauty and all the ways you may feel you fall short, you miss out on your own beauty.

- Your body design is a combination of traits inherited from your family.

- You have no *control* over the fact that you inherited Grandma's legs, Mom's waistline, and Dad's shoulders.

- You carry a small piece of all the people that went into creating you and who love you.

- Can you celebrate that fact?

- You may as well celebrate it since you *can't change it!*

- At some point in history, your body type *as it is today* was worshiped as the ideal.

- Even today, in spite of our culture, there are plenty of men who *love* larger, rounder, softer female bodies. And there are plenty of women who like massive men.

- Don't make the mistake of assuming that everyone prefers the same body type.

- There are people out there who would love and adore you and *your body*, *exactly* as you are now. Don't hide—advertise! And you'll find them!

Your body is *not* a design mistake.

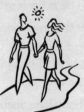

It is a *perfect* match for someone.

Be Willing to Heal at Your Own Pace

- If you broke a bone, would you compare notes with everyone else who broke that particular bone in order to determine how fast you were healing?

- Would you *judge* yourself harshly if you weren't healing as fast as someone else?

- No! That would be ridiculous!

- You would *accept* that your body has its own time line for healing.

- You might not *like* it, but you wouldn't *judge* yourself over it.

- Your spirit and body have their own time line for healing. You are *not in charge!*

- The biggest complaint we hear from others on their healing path is, "I should be further along than this."

- Who says? How do *you* know what recovery entails for you before you do it? You are like the farmer who pulls on the new shoots and says, "How come you aren't growing faster?"

- Don't resist—relax, accept, and know that you are growing as fast as you can!

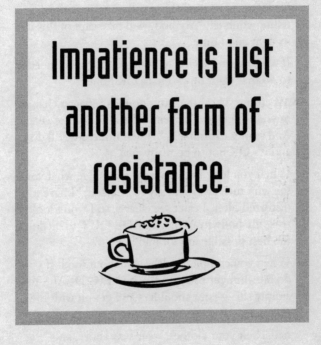

Impatience is just another form of resistance.

Recovery Is . . .

- When the pants you put on are too tight, you reach for leggings or something with an elastic waist, telling yourself, "My body will take care of this in its own good time."

- If you overate, saying to yourself, "I guess I needed to do that right now! That's OK honey."

- Accepting that those extra pounds reflect a change in your life that you aren't READY to make yet. And saying to yourself, "When I'm ready, I'll do it, and it's OK not to be ready yet!"

- When you look in the mirror and judge what you see, you turn away and say to yourself, "I have a distorted filter. I can't see clearly, so I won't look. I trust my body from the INSIDE OUT to be doing the best possible job for me!"

- When you completely RELAX about food. If you do non-hunger eating, IT'S NO BIG DEAL! You simply shrug your shoulders and get on with life!

- When you dress gorgeously, do your makeup, hair, nails, belt your clothes, wear sexy shoes, and lingerie, and flirt outrageously, no matter what your body size is!

The freedom to love food, love your body, and love life!

Listen to and Trust Yourself

- You didn't choose your personality. You were born with it.

- Every mother knows that her children are radically different from birth.

- You are a COMPLETELY UNIQUE physical, emotional, and spiritual being.

- There has never been, nor will there ever be, another you.

- You have unique gifts to offer this planet, but only if you are willing to discover them, claim them, and express them.

- This means, be willing to be yourself fully, no matter what others may think of you.

- God did not make a mistake designing you. You are a perfect creation.

- You are not a human being searching for spiritual answers.

- You are a spiritual being having a human experience. You have all of your answers within you, in your heart and your soul.

- Trust your body, trust your feelings, trust your heart, and trust yourself.

Your highest purpose is to be 100% yourself.

CHAPTER 12

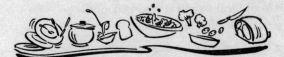

Questions
and
Answers

"What is my ideal weight?"

- Your ideal weight is your genetically predetermined setpoint.

- Your "setpoint" is determined from the inside out, not by the mirror.

- If you are eating only according to body hunger, and not overeating, your body will gradually melt down to your natural setpoint.

- How will you know when you have arrived at your genetic ideal weight?

  - *At your setpoint, you can eat a lot or a little and your weight won't change.*

  - *At your setpoint, you will feel light and energetic.*

  - *At your setpoint, you will feel great inside of your body.*

  - *At your setpoint, your weight varies from 5-10 lbs. It is not an exact number on the scale. The variation of 5-10 lbs. occurs depending on the time of the month, the season of the year, or your stress level. This is natural and normal.*

  - *At your setpoint, people will say, "You look fabulous!"*

At your setpoint, people will say, "You look fabulous," and you will *feel* fabulous inside your body.

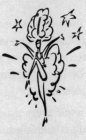

"But Every Time I Look in a Mirror, I Hate What I See."

- Once you acquire your ideal body, you may still have a distorted mind.

- If you have spent time and energy trying to reshape your body, chances are you have been trying to make it into something it can never be.

- Since our cultural ideal of a woman's body is a gross distortion, you end up with a distorted mental filter when you look at your own body because you compare it to what is unachievable for you and most people.

- A distorted mind cannot see its own ideal body with accuracy.

- Haven't you ever been as slim as you wanted to be and still were unhappy and dissatisfied with your body?

- Every mirror is different in terms of how fat or slim it makes you look. Since you have a distorted mental filter when you look at yourself anyway, counteract that by buying mirrors that make you look as slim as possible!

- And remind yourself every time you look in the mirror, "My body is melting into the best shape for me. I trust that it *will* show me what my ideal form and weight should be."

Buy slimming mirrors to counteract your distorted perception.

"Shall I Weigh Myself?"

- Throw out your scales today.

- We always weighed ourselves several times a day to try to keep our weight "under control."

- We discovered weighing ourselves only made us eat *more!*

  – *If we lost weight, we felt we had some leeway to eat.*

  – *If we gained weight, we ate because we were depressed.*

- Would you really *care* what the scale said if you had Christie Brinkley's body?

- The *number* on the scale tells you *nothing* about muscle mass, weight distribution, or tone. It tells you *nothing* about how you *look!*

- It just has the power to destroy your day!

- Weighing = giving your power to an outside authority and taking it away from an inner authority—your body.

- Weighing yourself only makes you fatter.

- Your body *knows* the ideal weight distribution for you. Allow yourself to discover it!

- Beating yourself up never made you slimmer.

- Also, cut all the size labels out of your clothes. Labels are just like the scales—another way you beat yourself up!

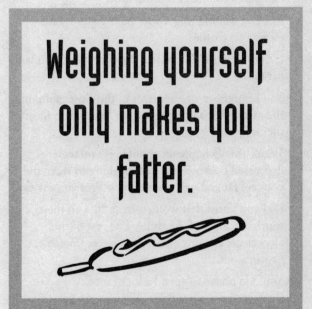

Weighing yourself
only makes you
fatter.

"I Don't Want to Buy New Clothes Until I'm Slimmer!"

- Dowdy clothes make you eat.

- What percentage of the clothes in your closet fit and make you feel beautiful now? _____ %

- Are you waiting to get slim before you spend money on clothes?

- It doesn't work! If you feel dowdy NOW, you will eat more!

- You keep those smaller sizes in the closet thinking they will *motivate* you to eat *less* in order to fit into them.

- What usually happens, though, is you feel depressed because you have nothing to wear and you feel fat and ugly—and that makes you eat *more!*

- Did you know that women wear 20% of their wardrobe 80% of the time? The rest of their clothes are either unflattering, uncomfortable, or worn out.[31]

- You don't have to spend a lot of money. Explore thrift stores in your town. You can get great finds in all sizes. Or, buy things you can belt or take in as you lose weight.

- Clean out your closet and go shopping.

- Pack away or give away anything in your closet that doesn't fit perfectly and make you feel gorgeous now!

Pack away or give away
anything in your closet
that doesn't fit perfectly
and make you feel
gorgeous now!

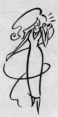

"I Just Overate; Now What?"

• It doesn't matter *at all* that you just overate. You were *not* bad and you *didn't* fail.

• Just *notice* how your body feels at this degree of fullness. What is that feeling like for you? Is it an experience you would enjoy repeating?

• Probably not, but it is an experience that you, like everyone else, will likely repeat again as you return to being a "normal eater." As long as you stay conscious, *without judgment*, you will become less and less willing to be uncomfortable.

• But right now, you're worried about those extra calories, right? *All* you have to do is wait until you are physically hungry to eat again—and any extra calories that you consumed will be burned off.

• The body doesn't send the hunger signal until it has *burned* all of the food from your last meal.

After overeating, just wait until you are physically hungry to eat again.

"Should I Tell My Friends What I'm Doing?"

- Tell only the ones you *know* will support you. Definitely enlist their support and share this book with them so they will understand what you are doing and how they can support you appropriately.

- Usually you get excited about a new way to eat and you run out and tell everyone! You are usually looking:

  – *for their support and approval.*

  – *for their agreement that you're doing the "right thing."*

  – *for converts—because that also validates that you made the right choice.*

  – *to justify why you are now eating fattening foods in front of them.*

- Instead of getting what you are looking for, you may get skepticism and disagreement because *everyone has an opinion* about what constitutes healthy or weight-loss eating!

- Some friends may *discourage* you or shoot you down. Let the changes in your weight and eating be your testimony.

- When you completely trust yourself to remain a "normal eater," then tell the world! (But *only* if they ask!)

- If you are working with a therapist, share this book so your therapist can also support you appropriately.

Don't worry about what *they* think.

Keep your eyes on your own paper.

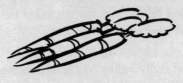

"How Do I Get 'My Share' Without Seeming Selfish?"

- At first, never share a meal, or if you do, divide it onto two separate plates. If you eat from the same plate, you may inhale your food to get "your share."

- You deserve to have foods you want available to you at all times. If you buy foods you want and your family eats them all before you get any, you aren't buying enough! Buy lots more, and make it a family rule that whoever eats the last of something needs to replace it or put it on the grocery list.

- Better yet, keep a hidden stash of foods you might want. Even if it's ice cream, you can put it into Tupperware containers and label it "gravy." Or wrap other things in aluminum foil in the fridge— and don't label or mislabel them.

- You need to know with absolute certainty that when you really want a cookie, the cookie will *be there!* If you don't get what you *really want* in that moment, you will probably overeat!

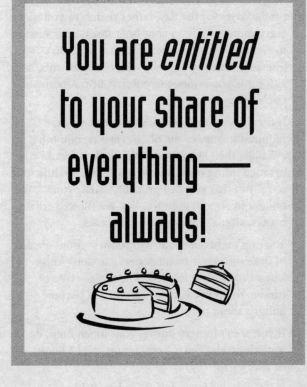

You are *entitled* to your share of everything— always!

"If I Eat Other Than at Lunchtime, My Boss Will Kill Me!"

- Most bosses are more concerned with your overall productivity for the day, rather than how you spend every minute. Talk to your boss and ask permission to eat on a flex-schedule, as long as it doesn't interfere with any of your work commitments, and as long as you arrange to cover your position while you're away.

- If that is *completely impossible*, because you are required to answer the phones at a certain time, for example, then keep food with you at work. As you practice eating consciously, it will take so little food to fill you that you will probably satisfy your hunger in 5 to 10 minutes. You *are* allowed coffee breaks, after all, and bathroom breaks.

- You don't schedule your bathroom sessions ahead of time with your boss because you don't know when they will be needed. The same is true of eating. You don't *know* when you will become hungry ahead of time.

- If you aren't hungry during your lunch hour, do something else fun. Go shopping, read a book, or take a nap!

- Keep a stash of wonderful food available at work so that you can eat whenever hunger hits.

Keep a stash of
wonderful food available
at work so you can eat
whenever hunger hits.

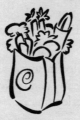

"Is There a Way to Make Sure I'm Hungry for a Lunch Date?"

- Yes. You can do what we call *PACING*.

- For example: Let's say you become hungry at 11:00 A.M.—and lunch is at 12:00. Do not try to wait until lunch because you will be too hungry and *will* overeat. Instead, have two bites of something, preferably protein, to take the edge off your hunger. Perhaps, two bites of cheese, or chicken, etc.

- *Do not* try to figure out how much food it's going to take to "hold you" until 12:00. It will invariably be too much.

- If your hunger comes back *again* before 12:00, have two more bites. But two bites *only*!

- In this way, you can make sure you are actually *hungry* at scheduled mealtimes. This will increase your pleasure greatly and make your body much happier than overloading it.

- Do not do the opposite of *PACING*, which is *PREVENTATIVE EATING* (i.e., eating before you are hungry so that hunger doesn't arrive at an inconvenient time).

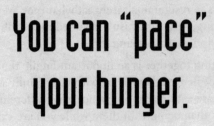

You can "pace" your hunger.

"How Do You Eat Only for Hunger with a Family?"

- If part of your responsibility in your family includes cooking the meals, begin to think of part of your job description as "chef!"

- Chefs in restaurants rarely eat what they are cooking. "Eating it" isn't included in the job description of "cooking it."

- If eating together is an important family time, go ahead! Be together! *Being* with your family while they are eating and you're not is no different for them than being with them while you are eating, too!

- The *social* part of the activity is the talking and the listening, not *watching* each other putting food in your mouths.

- Don't tell your family what you are doing— *just do it*. If they ask why you're not eating, you can truthfully say, "Oh, I'm not hungry," or "I had a late lunch and I'm stuffed."

- Or, if you prefer to eat together, practice "pacing." (See previous question.) Don't try to put your family on demand feeding, too.

- First become a normal eater, then the rest is easy!

Just because you cooked it doesn't mean you have to eat it!

"Don't I Have to Eat When Others Do in Order to be Sociable?"

- In our culture, we use eating as an excuse to spend time with people we like.

- Rather than just meeting to hang out, we meet over breakfast, lunch, dinner, or coffee.

- Simply because you meet in a restaurant doesn't mean you have to eat.

- You can order a drink, or even if you order food, don't eat it if you're not *hungry!* Have a bite or two, push it around on your plate, talk a lot, listen a lot, and ask for the rest to go!

- No one will even notice. They are usually too busy feeding themselves. *And* they will be flattered by your extra attentiveness.

The "social" part of social eating is the talking and listening— *not the eating.*

"I'm Afraid I'll be Judged if I Eat Something Fattening, Since I'm Not Slim!"

- Eating is as *personal* and as important as eliminating waste.

- Do you worry you'll be judged if you go to the bathroom as often as you need to?

- It is no one else's business *ever* what you do with food. It is completely between you and your body.

- Worrying about judgment from others has caused you to eat in secret, feel guilty, feel shame, and *eat more!*

- You are *entitled* to eat whatever you want in front of anyone.

- They don't need to know that you are *eating* your way to slimness.

- Don't apologize, don't explain.

- Just do it!

Do you worry you'll be judged if you go to the bathroom as often as you need to?

"Where Does Exercise Fit In?"

- What things do you love to do that involve movement?

- Make a list. Consider such things as dancing, gardening, walking on the beach, shopping, jumping rope, skipping. They all involve moving your body.

- You don't need to have a compulsive exercise regimen to be slim.

- But, your body is made of movable parts. It loves to move. Move it!

- You know this is true, because if you sit or lie down too long, you are stiff and creaky and your body shouts to be stretched and moved.

- Compulsive exercisers are very good at not listening to their bodies. They are determined to exercise the same amount (or more) every day, regardless of how their bodies feel about it! Some days you are stronger than others, some days weaker. Don't exercise according to an agenda. Listen to what your body wants.

- Move 12 minutes a day. No one is too busy to find 12 minutes a day to spend on movement!

- Your weight, however, is *primarily* a reflection of your eating. Exercise makes you fit and toned, but not necessarily slim.

Your body is made of movable parts.

It loves to move.

Move It!

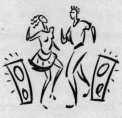

"I Feel Fat"

- If you are eating consciously, from hunger to satisfaction, you will *feel* light in your body.

- It is physically impossible to gain 10 lbs. overnight. If you're "feeling fat" today and yesterday you felt fine, chances are you are facing uncomfortable feelings that you'd rather avoid by focusing instead on how fat you feel!

- It's easier to focus on fat as the issue because, in the past, you thought that by dieting, you could do something about it.

- Now that you know fat is not the problem, you still may not be used to doing something about your uncomfortable feelings. Go back to Secret 7 and review how to focus on and take care of your true feeling and not the "fat" feeling.

- So anytime you "feel fat," ask yourself, "Did I just overeat?" If not, be a detective. Uncover and honor those uncomfortable feelings, and you will "feel fat" no more.

- "Feeling fat" only means you are avoiding some uncomfortable feelings.

"Feeling fat"
means you are
avoiding feelings.

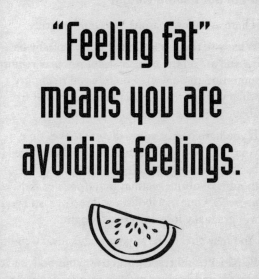

"I'm Eating Just Like You've Said, and I'm Not Losing Weight"

There are a few reasons this could be true:

1. What you think is a *2* and a *5* may actually be a *4* and a *7* on the hunger scale. You may require more fine-tuning. Are you *sure* you're hungry when you start? Is your approximate meal size about a fist size—or is it much more?

2. If you have been a yo-yo dieter, it takes time for your injured metabolism to heal and get raised back up to normal. This can take you from 8 to 14 months of normal eating. But, *if you just keep eating normally*, your metabolism will recover, and you will gradually lose any excess weight.

3. You may already be at your body's ideal weight.

Be patient, and respect and trust your body's natural hunger and healing process to give you your ideal body. Above all, enjoy your newfound power to enjoy eating.

Trust that your body's natural hunger will give you your ideal body.

If You Have More Questions

- Many questions not covered here will come up in the process of learning to trust your body.

- *Fortunately*, you don't have someone to ask what to do, because that would only take you further away from yourself.

- *No one* out there has the answers for exactly how you need to eat to have your best health and best body.

- But *your body knows*. All you have to do is keep consulting it.

- If your body feels pleasurable and comfortable, you are giving your body what it needs. If your body feels painful or uncomfortable, you are not listening to it.

- Your body was designed to motivate you to listen to it by making correct choices feel pleasurable and comfortable, and incorrect choices feel painful and uncomfortable.

- The only way you will discover what works best for you is through trial and error. Remember, no matter what you do, as long as you do it *consciously*, you will learn from it.

- Before long, you could write a book on *exactly* what makes your body feel great. You will have discovered your own answers, and in the process you will have learned that you and your body are completely trustworthy.

- Trust your body, trust your feelings, trust yourself. That's all there is.

Trust your body.
Trust your feelings.
Trust yourself.
That's all there is!

Hunger Rating Scale

0– *You are starving.*

1– *Too hungry to care* what you eat.

2– *SERIOUSLY HUNGRY. Your body is sending unmistakable messages that it* must *eat* now.

3– *Moderately hungry.* You could wait another twenty minutes.

4– *Slightly hungry.* You could eat, but you could also wait.

5– *COMFORTABLE.* You are no longer aware of being hungry or of any sense of fullness or sensation of food in your stomach. You *could* put your plate aside and wait 30 minutes before finishing. At a 5, notice that your food *begins* to taste like cardboard. If you are not sure that you are at a 5, take 3 bites of the best thing on your plate and check again.

TEAR ALONG PERFORATED LINE

The Seven Secrets of Slim People

1) Listen to your *body*, not your *mind*.

2) Eat *with* awareness, and *without* judgment.

3) Eat only when you are *physically* hungry.

4) Stop eating when you are *satisfied*, not *full*.

5) Eat what you want most.

6) Notice how your body feels *after* eating.

7) *Honor* your feelings; don't bury them under food.

Hunger Rating Scale

6– *Slightly uncomfortable*. You are aware of feeling food in your stomach.

7– *Uncomfortable*. Sleepy, sluggish, tired, you feel full.

8– *Very uncomfortable*. Stomach hurts and you yearn to lay down.

9– *Stuffed*. You feel like a sausage.

10– *So stuffed* you have to be wheeled away from the table in a wheelbarrow.

TEAR ALONG PERFORATED LINE

Using the Non-Hunger Eating Urge as a Doorway to Feeding Emotional Hungers

1) Ask yourself: "Am I physically hungry?"

2) If the answer is no, ask yourself: "What am I really hungry for?"

3) Ask yourself: "What baby step can I take right now to give myself a little bit of what I really want?"

4) DO IT!

5) If it takes more than 15 minutes or more than $15 it is not a baby step.

Endnotes

1. *Life* magazine, February 1995, "28 Questions about Fat." p.62.

2. United States Surgeon General's Annual Report, Fall, 1995.

3. 1996 Council on Size and Weight Discrimination, Inc. PO Box 305, Mt. Marion, NY 12456. (Reprinted with permission).

4. *People* magazine, "Too Fat? Too Thin?", June 3, 1996, p. 71.

5. Keys, A., Brozek, J., Henschel, A., Mickelsen, O., & Taylor, H.L. (1950). *The biology of human starvation.* Minneapolis: University of Minnesota Press.

6. Ibid.

7. Ibid.

8. Roth, Geenen. (1984). *Breaking Free from Compulsive Eating.* New York: Signet.

9. Pearson, L., Pearson, L. (1973) *The Psychologist's Eat-Anything Diet.* New York: Peter H 179 Publishers, p. 250.

10. Boyle, P.C., Storlien, H., & Keesey, R.E. (1978). Increased efficiency of food utilization following weight loss. *Physiology and Behavior,* 21, 261.

11. *People* magazine, June 3, 1996, "Too Fat? Too Thin?" p.67.

12. Ibid. p.67.

13. Ibid. p.67.

14. Ibid. p.66.

15. Ibid. p.66.

16. Keys, A., Brozek, J., Henschel, A., Mickelsen, O., & Taylor, H.L. (1950). *The biology of human starvation.* Minneapolis: University of Minnesota Press.

17. Groger, Molly. (1983) *Eating Awareness Training,* New York: Summit Books.

18. *San Luis Obispo Telegram-Tribune,* April 22, 1996, D-4.

19. Herman, C.P. and Mack, D. (1975) "Restrained and Unrestrained Eating." *Journal of Personality,* vol. 43, p. 647-660.

20. Bennet, W., & Gurin, J. (1982). *The dieter's dilemma: Eating less and weighing more*. New York: Basic Books.

21. Sims, E.A.H., Goldman, R., Gluck, C., Horton, E.S., Kelleher, P., & Rowe, D. (1968). Experimental obesity in man. *Transcript of the Association of American Physicians*, 81, 153.

22. Schwartz, Bob. (1982). *Diets Don't Work*. Las Vegas: Breakthru Publishing.

23. Groger, Molly. (1983). *Eating Awareness Training*.

24. Shaevitz, Mort. (1994). *Lean and Mean*.

25. Ribble, Margaret. *The Rights of Infants*. and Spock, Benjamin. *Baby and Child Care*.

26. Mumma, J.D. Myth: "Sumo Wrestlers eat all day," *Living Better magazine*, 1996, vol. 4 #2, p. 28.

27. Roth, Geneen. (1984). *Breaking Free from Compulsive Eating*. New York: Signet.

28. Kunz, Mary, MFCC Intern. (1996) "Baby Steps, Miracle Growth." Class Lecture, EAT-SLO, eating disorders program.

29. Latimer, Jane Evans. (1990). *Living Binge Free*. Colorado: Living Quest.

30. Roth, Geneen.

31. *Good Housekeeping*, June 1996, p. 141.

For More Information:

1-800-777-5613
PERSONAL TELEPHONE SUPPORT

Everyone benefits from the support of personal attention. We provide Personal Telephone Support to help you make the transition from overeating to total freedom with food. Skilled experts who have had long-term success with The Seven Secrets method will tailor a program to your specific needs, working with you by phone, anywhere in the country. They will compassionately guide you through your fears and individual obstacles, enabling you to become permanently free from food or weight problems.

Call for your *free* initial consultation!

Form Your Own Support Group

When we first began changing from overeaters to normal eaters, we started our own support group with others who wanted to make the same change. Practicing the Seven Secrets method with others made the change easy and enjoyable. We are happy to help you start you own support group or join one already existing in your area.

Support Group Kits

The Support Group Kits will do all the work for you. Please call us at our toll-free phone number for more information.

Seminars and Speaking Engagements

We invite you to join the many others who sponsor or participate in our seminars, workshops, and lectures. We tailor our presentations to the special needs of your audience, be it corporate, charity, spiritual, educational, or political. Above all, we are dedicated to meeting the unique needs of you and the audience.

Web Site Address

You may also reach us at:
http://members.aol.com/t7secret/index.html

Reader Response Card

PLEASE TAKE ADVANTAGE OF OUR SPECIAL OFFER!

1. COMMENTS: We care greatly about our readers and often speak with them directly. We would love your feedback on *The Seven Secrets of Slim People*. Please write us your comments below:

2. SPECIAL OFFER WITH THIS CARD: Send back this card and we are happy to give you the following special offer:

   A set of 4 audio tapes, 60 minutes each, that go along with this book and make even easier your personal freedom from food and weight. They contain additional examples and information not found in the book. They are a great reinforcement.

   Regular price $39.95   *Special Offer With This Card Only:* $19.95

3. Mail in this card for a free catalog of audio tapes and to receive our free quarterly newsletter.

4. Also, please call me for a free personal telephone consultation. The best phone numbers and times to reach me are: _____

5. Name: _____
   Address: _____
   Phone: _____